Introduction

Sometimes, the strength of motherhood is greater than natural laws.

Barbara Kingsolver

Becoming a mother is one of life's most incredible journeys, filled with so much love, happiness, and a sense of completeness that you've never felt before. However, it's no secret that this life-changing experience also comes with its fair share of challenges. I am not just talking about the physical recovery we face post-childbirth but also the emotional rollercoaster that follows. Motherhood can often feel completely overwhelming, especially when coupled with the societal pressures we face as new parents and even our own personal expectations.

You picked up this book, so I'm assuming you can relate. As a new mom, you may find yourself grappling with a vast array of difficulties. Recovering from the physical toll of childbirth, navigating the steep learning curve of infant care, and managing the emotional upheaval can all contribute to feelings of exhaustion, self-doubt, and even a sense of isolation. Right now, you may be questioning your ability to be a good mother, struggling with body image issues, or feeling like you've lost touch with your pre-baby self.

The first thing I want you to know is this: **These challenges, no matter how daunting they may seem, are a normal part of the motherhood journey.**

And here's the good news: You don't have to face these trials alone!

Self-care, although often overlooked, is a powerful tool that can help you navigate the postpartum period with more ease, resilience, and confidence. By prioritizing your own well-being, you can cultivate the strength and serenity needed to fully embrace your role as a mother.

As a mother of three who has navigated the postpartum journey myself, I understand firsthand the challenges and triumphs that come during this time. When I first became a mother, I found myself struggling to balance the demands of caring for my baby with my own physical and emotional needs. I felt overwhelmed, exhausted, and, at times, isolated in my struggles.

It was through my own journey of self-discovery and healing that I realized the immense power of self-care in the postpartum period. As I sank my teeth into research and connected with other mothers, I discovered that there was a

THE PRACTICAL GUIDE TO POSTPARTUM SELF-CARE

A Holistic Approach to Transform Your Physical,
Emotional, and Mental Well-Being

AVA WELLS

Table of Contents

Introduction   5

Part I: Embracing the Change

1. Embracing New Beginnings—The Journey Into
   Motherhood   13

Part II: Physical Well-Being

2. Nourishing New Life—Mastering Postpartum
   Nutrition   29
3. Rest and Rejuvenation—Finding Peace in
   Postpartum Sleep   45
4. Regaining Strength—Postpartum Exercise and
   Wellness   55
5. Nurturing Breast and Vaginal Health
   Postpartum   71

Part III: Emotional and Mental Well-Being

6. Serenity in Motherhood—Managing Stress
   After Birth   91
7. Beyond the Blues—Understanding Postpartum
   Depression   107
8. Body Image and Self-Confidence in
   Motherhood   123

Part IV: Bonding With Baby

9. Gentle Beginnings—Essentials of Newborn
   Bonding   139

Part V: Thriving as a Woman and a Mom

10. Building Your Village—Nurturing Connections
    in Motherhood   159
11. Harmonizing Life—Balancing Motherhood
    With Personal Growth   169

Conclusion   179
References   183

wealth of knowledge and practical strategies out there that helped me to truly thrive as a new mom.

Inspired by my own experiences and driven by a passion to support other mothers, I set out to write this book. My goal is to create a resource that offers the guidance, encouragement, and practical tools I wish I had during those early days of motherhood. I want to empower *you* with evidence-based strategies and heartfelt wisdom so you can approach this chapter of life with more confidence, self-compassion, and resilience.

Throughout this book, I'll be sharing not only my own insights but also the collective wisdom of countless mothers who have walked this path before you. I hope that by offering a blend of scientific research and the lived experiences of real mothers, you'll find the support and validation you need to prioritize your own well-being.

Above all, I want you to know that you are not alone in this journey. By shining a light on the common struggles and joys of mothers, I hope to help you find a sense of community and connection. Together, we can challenge the insane narrative that self-care is selfish and instead embrace it as an essential part of our motherhood journey.

So, as you read through these pages, know that I am here with you, cheering you on every step of the way. Let this book be a reminder that you deserve to prioritize your own well-being and that by doing so, you're not only caring for yourself and your baby but also laying the foundation for a more joyful and fulfilling motherhood experience.

Here are some of the things we're going to cover:

- nourishing your body with proper nutrition
- finding moments of rest and rejuvenation amid the chaos
- rebuilding physical strength through gentle exercise
- fostering a positive body image and self-confidence
- nurturing your bond with your baby
- creating a supportive network
- finding harmony between your identity as a mother and as an individual

When you take the steps to care for your own needs, you will find that you have more energy, patience, and presence to offer your baby and your loved ones. You'll be better equipped to handle the inevitable challenges and savor all those precious moments of connection and growth. People aren't kidding when they say if you blink, you'll miss it! This precious time with your new baby won't last very long. In order to make the most of it, you really need to be present and available—two things that are impossible when you're dysregulated, stressed, and exhausted.

You deserve to enjoy your role as a mother, not just survive. And your baby deserves an engaged mama who is not stuck in survival mode. So, congratulations on taking this first step toward prioritizing your well-being. You're here, reading this book, so you're already demonstrating the strength, wisdom, and love that will guide you through this incredible journey.

As you work through the pages ahead, know that you are part of a community of mothers who are all navigating their own unique paths yet sharing similar struggles, triumphs, and aspirations. By embracing self-care and leaning into the support of others, I promise that you'll discover reserves of resilience and joy you never even knew you had.

Remember: Caring for yourself is an essential part of caring for your baby. So, take a deep breath, trust your innate strength, and set aside this outdated notion that mothers simply have to *endure* and keep going. Your journey to a more nourished, empowered, fulfilled, and *purposeful* motherhood starts right now!

Part I: Embracing the Change

Embracing New Beginnings—The Journey Into Motherhood

I like to think of motherhood as a great big adventure. You set off on a journey, you don't really know how to navigate things, and you don't exactly know where you're going or how you're going to get there.

Cynthia Rowley

The path to motherhood really is a great adventure filled with excitement, uncertainty, and a whole host of changes that continue to unfold long after the birth of your little one. From the moment you hold your newborn in your arms, you find yourself stepping into a new role that will forever redefine your identity and reshape your world. This chapter is dedicated to guiding you through the emotional and physical changes that accompany the early stages of motherhood, offering support, understanding, and practical insights to help you embrace these new beginnings with confidence and grace.

It's so important to recognize that the changes you experience are not limited to the nine months of pregnancy or the intense moments of childbirth, although this might be all you have thought about for the last nine months! The journey of motherhood is an ongoing process of growth, adaptation, and self-discovery that extends well beyond the postpartum period.

Throughout this chapter, we will explore the various facets of this incredible transition, from the emotional highs and lows to the physical recovery and the shifting dynamics of your relationships. We'll discuss the importance of self-care, the power of a supportive network, and the strategies for navigating the challenges that may arise along the way.

Adjusting Your Mindset

As you set out on the journey of motherhood, it's crucial to recognize the significant role your mindset plays in shaping the whole experience for you. Cultivating a healthy and adaptable mindset can help you navigate the ups and downs of this phase of your life with greater resilience and self-compassion.

One key strategy is to **set realistic expectations for yourself and your motherhood journey**. Holding onto unrealistic standards or perfectionist ideals can lead to disappointment, guilt, and shame. Instead, you can allow yourself room for growth and learning by embracing the idea that motherhood is messy, imperfect, and full of surprises. This way, you create a more supportive and forgiving environment for yourself.

Another essential aspect of preparing mentally for motherhood is to **approach your birth and postpartum plans with flexibility.** While it's important to have preferences and goals in anything in life, holding onto a rigid plan can set you up for severe disappointment when things don't go as envisioned. Embrace the concept of "planning for the unplanned" by considering various possible outcomes and focusing on the aspects you can control instead of the ones you can't. For example, you can control your mindset and self-care practices, but you can't control when your baby starts to sleep through the night.

Above all, remember to **practice self-compassion** throughout your motherhood journey. Treat yourself with the same kindness, understanding, and forgiveness you would offer to a dear friend. Acknowledge that you are doing your best and that it's okay to have moments of struggle or uncertainty.

You can change your whole experience of motherhood by simply adjusting your mindset in these small but powerful ways, allowing for a much more positive and empowering experience.

Embracing the New Role

Now, don't panic, but this needs to be said here: Becoming a mother changes you fundamentally—in the most beautiful ways! This is a journey of personal growth and self-discovery that reshapes your identity, priorities, and perspective.

One of the most significant changes you may experience is a **heightened sense of protectiveness** toward your child. As a mother, you develop an instinctive drive to safeguard your baby from harm, both physically and emotionally. This fierce love and dedication become a guiding force in your life, influencing your decisions and actions.

Motherhood also teaches you **the art of adaptability**. As you navigate the ever-changing needs of your baby, you learn to adjust to new routines, challenges, and priorities. You become more flexible, resilient, and resourceful, discovering inner strengths you may not have even known you already possessed.

Along with this newfound strength, motherhood can also make you **feel more vulnerable**. The depth of love you feel for your child can be both exhilarating and frightening as you realize the immense responsibility of nurturing and shaping another life. This vulnerability, however, is also a source of growth, as it opens you up to new levels of empathy, compassion, and emotional depth.

As a mother, you may find that your **instincts become sharper and more attuned to your baby's needs**. You develop a unique bond with your child, learning to interpret their cues and respond with loving care. This heightened intuition extends beyond your role as a mother, enhancing your ability to read and connect with others in your life; it's a powerful skill, bringing new levels of joy and awareness to your life.

Perhaps one of the most profound changes motherhood brings is a **shift in priorities**. Your focus naturally gravitates toward your child's well-being, and you may find yourself reevaluating what truly matters in life. The things that once seemed important may pale in comparison to the joy and fulfillment of nurturing your baby.

It's important to honor these changes, not hide from them. There will be times when things are more challenging than before. Remembering that you are growing, learning, and developing new skills as your baby does the same will help you to have grace for yourself instead of doubting yourself. Remember, all moms experience these changes differently, so you may not experience these right away—that's completely normal! Each journey is unique.

Physical Changes

Obviously, carrying a child in your womb for nine months is going to change you physically. Your stomach expanding is probably the most well-known change of motherhood! But I want to talk to you about the other kinds of physical changes you can expect because understanding these changes and how to manage them can help you navigate this time with greater comfort and confidence.

Temporary Changes

In the early days and weeks following delivery, you may experience a range of temporary physical symptoms (Cleveland Clinic, 2018; March of Dimes, n.d.-b):

- If you had a cesarean section, you might notice some incision discharge as your wound heals.

- Your breasts may also produce discharge, become engorged, or feel tender as your milk supply establishes itself.
- Discomfort in the perineal area is common, especially if you had a vaginal delivery or required stitches.
- As your uterus shrinks back to its pre-pregnancy size, you may feel contractions, often referred to as afterpains. These contractions can be particularly noticeable during breastfeeding.
- You might also experience urination contractions, incontinence, or constipation as your pelvic floor muscles regain strength.
- Increased perspiration is another common postpartum symptom, as your body works to regulate its hormones and fluid levels.

To manage these physical changes, practice good hygiene, wear supportive garments, and use ice packs or warm compresses for comfort. Engage in pelvic floor exercises to rebuild strength and control. Stay hydrated, eat a balanced diet rich in fiber, and get plenty of rest to support your body's healing process.

Long-Lasting Changes

In addition to the temporary changes, pregnancy and child-birth can also lead to some long-lasting or permanent physical transformations. You may not experience any of these, or you may experience some of them. It's important to have an idea of what to expect either way (*6 Body Changes After Pregnancy*, n.d.; Hagen, 2018; Migala, 2023).

- Your alcohol sensitivity may increase, and your breasts may change in size, shape, or texture.
- Some women experience changes in their fingers, such as swelling or altered sensitivity.
- Your foot size and structure might also shift, requiring new shoes.
- Hormonal fluctuations can cause hair changes, such as temporary hair loss or altered texture.
- Your hips may widen, and the linea nigra, the dark line that appeared on your abdomen during pregnancy, may persist for some time.
- Your menstrual cycle will also gradually resume, though it may take several weeks or months to establish a regular pattern, especially if you are breastfeeding.

All of the physical changes you have experienced are a testament to the incredible journey of bringing new life into this world. Be patient and kind to yourself as you heal and adapt to your new postpartum body. If any symptoms persist or cause concern, don't hesitate to reach out to your healthcare provider for guidance and support.

Emotional Changes

The postpartum period is a time of significant emotional upheaval as new mothers navigate the complex and often overwhelming feelings that come with the transition into motherhood. After giving birth, you may experience a wide range of emotions, from elation and joy to unrest, anxiety, and even depression.

In the initial days after delivery, many mothers feel a profound sense of elation and euphoria. This heightened emotional state is characterized by intense feelings of love, empathy, and connection with your newborn. However, these positive emotions can quickly give way to feelings of unrest, often referred to as the "**baby blues**," as the reality of caring for a new baby sets in.

You may find yourself feeling **more alert and vigilant**, constantly attuned to your baby's needs. This heightened state of awareness can be both emotionally and physically taxing. Some mothers also experience unexpected feelings of aggression or irritability as the demands of motherhood and the lack of sleep take their toll.

For some women, the postpartum period can also bring about **feelings of disappointment or sadness**. You may feel disconnected from your pre-baby self or struggle with the idea that motherhood isn't exactly what you expected. In more severe cases, postpartum depression can develop, characterized by persistent feelings of sadness, hopelessness, and difficulty bonding with your baby.

The postpartum period is emotionally turbulent due to a complex interplay of hormonal changes, sleep deprivation, and the overwhelming responsibility of caring for a new life. The rapid drop in estrogen and progesterone levels after childbirth can contribute to **mood swings and emotional vulnerability**.

Just as with the physical changes, it's essential to remember that these emotional changes are a *normal* part of the postpartum experience. Be gentle with yourself and reach out for support when needed. Share your feelings with your partner, family, or friends, and don't hesitate to seek professional help if you find yourself struggling with persistent or severe emotional difficulties.

Why Self-Care?

Self-care is the practice of taking intentional actions to promote one's physical, mental, and emotional well-being. It involves nurturing yourself, setting boundaries, and prioritizing your needs to maintain a healthy and balanced life (Global Self-Care Federation, n.d.). In the context of motherhood, self-care becomes even more crucial, especially during the postpartum period.

As a new mother, you are faced with the overwhelming responsibility of caring for a tiny, dependent human being. The demands of motherhood can easily overshadow your own needs, leaving you feeling depleted, stressed, and emotionally drained (Geisinger, n.d.). However, neglecting self-care can have serious consequences, not only for your own well-being but also for your ability to care for your baby.

Throughout this book, we will emphasize the importance of self-care for mothers, making it our top priority. We will explore practical strategies and techniques to help you integrate self-care into your daily life, even amid the chaos of early motherhood. We will remind you that self-care doesn't need to be expensive or time-consuming and we'll encourage you to only use the strategies that resonate with you (just forget about the rest!). We will also prepare you to expect some very challenging days when it won't feel possible to fit in self-care. And we will challenge you to consider that those may be the days you need it most.

Think of the common analogy of putting on your own oxygen mask first before assisting others during an emergency on an airplane. As humans, we all have "oxygen masks" in our own lives: our energy, time, and resources. By filling your own tank first, you ensure that you have the capacity to nurture and care for your baby.

When you prioritize self-care, whether it's through nourishing your body with healthy food, getting enough sleep, or engaging in physical activity, you replenish your energy reserves. This, in turn, allows you to show up as the best version of yourself for your baby and your loved ones.

Remember, it is not selfish to prioritize taking care of yourself. It is essential to embrace self-care. When you do this, you are not only investing in your own health and happiness but also in your ability to be a present, patient, and loving mother to your child.

Starting the Self-Care Journey With a Journal

I know what you're thinking—what mom has time for journaling? But even a few minutes a week can help! Journaling can be a very powerful tool during your self-care journey. Creating and maintaining a journal can provide you with a sacred space for self-reflection, emotional processing, and goal setting. There are many ways to journal, so experiment and choose a journaling method that appeals to you. Feel free to change it up anytime, depending on what feels right for you. Here are some considerations before getting started:

- **Choose your journal format and technique:** Decide whether you prefer a traditional pen and paper journal or a digital format. Also, consider various journaling techniques such as free writing, gratitude journaling, or one-line-a-day journaling. Select a journal that resonates with you and inspires you to write.
- **Set aside dedicated time:** Try to establish a regular journaling routine by carving out a few minutes each day for self-reflection. Choose a time that works best for you but keep expectations realistic—there will be days when you need to be more flexible. If every day seems daunting, aim for once a week or any time frame that doesn't stress you out.
- **Create a conducive environment:** Find a quiet, comfortable space where you can write with minimal distractions. Light a candle, play soft music, or make a cup of tea to enhance the ambiance.
- **Start with self-reflective prompts:** Consider beginning each journaling session with a prompt that encourages introspection and self-discovery. Prompts are a useful tool to help spark inspiration and simply begin writing. Here are five prompts to get you started:

  - What are three things I'm grateful for today, and why?

- ○ What emotions have I been experiencing lately, and how can I navigate them in a healthy way?
- ○ What does self-care mean to me, and how can I incorporate more of it into my daily life?
- ○ What are my top priorities in this season of motherhood, and how can I align my actions with these priorities?
- ○ What is one small step I can take today to nurture my mind, body, or spirit?

- **Write freely and without judgment:** Allow your thoughts and feelings to flow onto the page without censoring yourself. Embrace the process of self-discovery and resist the urge to edit or critique your writing.
- **Reflect and revisit:** After each journaling session, take a moment to reflect on what you've written. Notice any patterns, insights, or areas for growth. Revisit your journal entries regularly to track your progress and celebrate your successes.
- **Let go of the pressure:** Journaling is not meant to be just another item on your to-do list. Try to take the pressure off and remain open to journaling when it feels right for you – if that time never comes or you discover journaling isn't your thing, that's perfectly okay. Only you know what's best for you.
- **Consider privacy:** If you feel uncomfortable leaving your unfiltered thoughts exposed in a journal that someone could read, consider the different privacy options available. You could write in your journal, and if you prefer to keep it private,

store it in a locked safe. Or, if you write digitally, you might keep it private with password protection and encryption. Some people feel better destroying or deleting their journal entries when finished but be sure to think twice before you do this; it is your story and your truth, and you may want to look back on it someday.

Your journal is a safe and private space where you can explore your innermost thoughts and feelings. Consider using it as a tool for self-care, self-discovery, and personal growth.

Key Takeaways and What's Next

In this chapter, we explored the different emotional and physical changes that accompany the journey into motherhood. We discussed the importance of adjusting your mindset, embracing your new role, and understanding the various physical and emotional transformations you may experience during the postpartum period.

Remember, prioritizing your well-being is crucial for navigating this time in your life. When you can understand and manage the physical changes after pregnancy, you are setting yourself up for a healthier and more balanced postpartum experience. Engage in self-care practices, seek support when needed, and be patient and compassionate with yourself as you adapt to your new reality.

We also introduced the concept of journaling as a powerful self-care tool. By creating a dedicated space for self-reflection and emotional processing, you can foster greater self-awareness, set intentions, and track your progress on your self-care journey.

As you move forward, commit to prioritizing self-care as an essential part of your motherhood journey. Use your journal to explore your thoughts, feelings, and experiences and to set small, achievable goals for nurturing your well-being.

We're now moving into Part 2, which looks closely at your physical well-being. We'll begin by discussing the importance of nutrition and diet for postpartum care. We'll explore how nourishing your body with the right foods can support your recovery, promote healing, and enhance your overall well-being.

Part II: Physical Well-Being

TWO

Nourishing New Life—Mastering Postpartum Nutrition

Our body is the only one we've been given, so we need to maintain it; we need to give it the best nutrition.

Trudie Styler

Your body really is a precious gift that deserves the best care and nourishment. This is especially true during the postpartum period, when your body undergoes significant changes and requires optimal nutrition to heal, recover, and support the demands of motherhood.

Postpartum nutrition can feel overwhelming, particularly when navigating motherhood for the first time. With so much information available and the pressure to "bounce back" after pregnancy, it's easy to feel lost or confused about what to eat and how to properly fuel your body. It's also really easy to neglect yourself in the chaos of having a new baby.

In this chapter, I am going to guide you through the essentials of postpartum nutrition, providing you with the knowledge and tools to make informed choices that support your recovery, promote milk production (if breastfeeding), and enhance your overall well-being. We'll explore the importance of key nutrients, discuss calorie intake changes, and offer practical tips for creating a balanced and nourishing postpartum diet.

Remember that this is a time to be gentle with yourself and honor the incredible work your body has done in bringing new life into the world. Rather than focusing on restrictive diets or rapid weight loss, my goal is to empower you with the information and strategies to make nutritious choices that support your unique needs and promote a healthy, sustainable recovery.

Importance of Nutrition for Postpartum Care

Proper nutrition is so important in the postpartum period, as it supports the mother's recovery, promotes milk production (if breastfeeding), and contributes to overall well-being. Your postpartum nutrition lays the foundation for a healthy and successful transition into motherhood.

Firstly, a well-balanced postpartum diet can **significantly speed up your recovery process**. During pregnancy and childbirth, your body undergoes tremendous physical strain and requires essential nutrients to heal and rebuild. Consuming a variety of nutrient-dense foods, such as lean proteins, whole grains, fruits, and vegetables, provides your body with the building blocks it needs to repair tissues, reduce inflammation, and promote healing (Chen et al., 2018).

Moreover, if you choose to breastfeed, postpartum nutrition is crucial for **maintaining an adequate milk supply**. Breastfeeding places additional nutritional demands on the mother's body, as it requires extra energy and nutrients to produce breast milk (NHS, n.d.). Consuming a balanced diet that includes plenty of protein, calcium, and fluids helps ensure that your body has the resources it needs to produce high-quality, nutritious breast milk for your growing baby.

Beyond physical recovery and milk production, postpartum nutrition also plays a significant role in **supporting your overall well-being**. The postpartum period can be physically and emotionally demanding, and proper nutrition can help you maintain energy levels, stabilize your mood, and promote mental clarity. Consuming a diet rich in whole foods, healthy fats, and complex carbohydrates can help keep your blood sugar levels stable, reducing the likelihood of experiencing energy crashes or mood swings (Firth et al., 2020).

It's important to note that your calorie intake needs will change during the postpartum period, particularly if you are breastfeeding. On average, breastfeeding mothers require an additional 500 calories per day to support milk production and maintain their own health (National Institute of Health, n.d.). However, it's essential to focus on the *quality* of those additional calories, choosing nutrient-dense foods that provide a balance of protein, calcium, and other essential nutrients.

Remember, every mother's nutritional needs are unique, and it's crucial to listen to your body's cues and adjust your diet accordingly. Consult with your healthcare provider or a registered dietitian to develop a personalized postpartum nutrition plan that takes into account your specific needs, preferences, and dietary restrictions.

When you prioritize postpartum nutrition, you're investing in your own health and well-being and providing the best possible start for your baby. Nourishing your body with the right foods can make a significant difference in your recovery, milk production, and overall sense of vitality during this time of your life.

Nutrients for New Moms

As a new mom, ensuring that you're getting the right nutrients is crucial for your health and the health of your baby, especially if you're breastfeeding. Let's take a closer look at some of the top nutrients needed for postpartum care.

Protein

- **Description:** Protein is an essential macronutrient that plays a vital role in rebuilding and repairing tissues, producing hormones and enzymes, and supporting immune function.
- **Purpose:** Adequate protein intake is crucial for postpartum recovery, as it helps heal tissues damaged during childbirth and supports the production of breast milk.

- **Recommended daily intake:** Breastfeeding mothers need about 25 grams more protein per day than non-pregnant women, which equates to a total of 71 grams of protein daily (Wati et al., 2023).
- **Food sources:** Lean meats, poultry, fish, eggs, dairy products, legumes, nuts, and seeds.

Calcium

- **Description:** Calcium is a mineral that is essential for building and maintaining strong bones and teeth.
- **Purpose:** During lactation, calcium is crucial for maintaining the mother's bone density and supporting the baby's growing skeletal system.
- **Recommended daily intake:** Breastfeeding mothers need 1,000 mg of calcium per day (Nemours KidsHealth, n.d.).
- **Food sources:** Dairy products, leafy green vegetables, calcium-fortified foods, and supplements.

Iron

- **Description:** Iron is a mineral that is essential for the production of hemoglobin, a protein in red blood cells that carries oxygen throughout the body.
- **Purpose:** Many women experience iron deficiency anemia after childbirth due to blood loss during delivery. Adequate iron intake helps replenish iron stores and prevent anemia.
- **Recommended daily intake:** Postpartum women need 9 mg of iron per day, while breastfeeding

mothers need 10 mg (*Can a Mother Be Iron-Deficient While Breastfeeding?* n.d.).

- **Food sources:** Red meat, poultry, fish, iron-fortified cereals, dark leafy greens, and legumes.

Vitamin B12

- **Description:** Vitamin B12 is a water-soluble vitamin that plays a crucial role in red blood cell formation, neurological function, and DNA synthesis.
- **Purpose:** Adequate vitamin B12 intake is important for maintaining energy levels, supporting neurological development in infants, and preventing anemia.
- **Recommended daily intake:** Breastfeeding mothers need 2.8 mcg of vitamin B12 per day (Vitamin B12, 2024).
- **Food sources:** Animal products such as meat, fish, poultry, eggs, and dairy. Fortified plant-based foods and supplements are options for vegetarians and vegans.

DHA

- **Description:** DHA is an omega-3 fatty acid that is important for brain and eye development in infants.
- **Purpose:** Adequate DHA intake supports the cognitive and visual development of breastfed infants and may have benefits for maternal mental health.
- **Recommended daily intake:** Breastfeeding

mothers should aim for 200–300 mg of DHA per day (Juber et al., 2016).

- **Food sources:** Fatty fish, like salmon, sardines, and anchovies. Algae-based supplements are available for vegetarians and vegans.

Choline

- **Description:** Choline is an essential nutrient that plays a role in brain development, liver function, and metabolism.
- **Purpose:** Adequate choline intake during lactation supports the cognitive development of infants and may have long-term benefits for their memory and learning abilities.
- **Recommended daily intake:** Breastfeeding mothers need 550 mg of choline per day (CDC, 2024).
- **Food sources:** Eggs, beef liver, chicken, fish, cruciferous vegetables, and soybeans.

Vitamin D

- **Description:** Vitamin D is a fat-soluble vitamin that is important for calcium absorption, immune function, and bone health.
- **Purpose:** Adequate vitamin D intake is crucial for maintaining maternal bone health and supporting the healthy development of the baby's skeletal system.

- **Recommended daily intake:** Breastfeeding mothers need 15 mcg (600 IU) of vitamin D per day (La Leche League International, n.d.).
- **Food sources:** Fatty fish, egg yolks, fortified dairy products, and supplements. Sun exposure also helps the body synthesize vitamin D.

Remember, while focusing on these key nutrients, it's essential to consume a well-rounded, balanced diet that includes a variety of nutrient-dense foods. If you have specific concerns or dietary restrictions, consult with your healthcare provider or a registered dietitian to ensure you're meeting your individual nutritional needs.

Postpartum Diet

Navigating your postpartum diet can be overwhelming, especially with the added responsibility of caring for a newborn. However, making informed choices about your nutrition can really help to support your recovery and overall well-being. Let's explore some postpartum diet guidelines and the best foods to eat during this time (Lindberg, 2020b; Parker, 2022; *Postpartum Diet and Weight Loss*, n.d; Traxler, 2023):

Postpartum Diet Guidelines

- Choose a wide variety of foods from all food groups to ensure you're getting a balance of essential nutrients.
- Stay hydrated throughout the day by drinking plenty of water and other healthy fluids.

- Keep an eye on your calorie intake, ensuring you're consuming enough to support recovery and milk production (if breastfeeding) without going overboard.
- Remember that postpartum weight loss should be slow and gradual. Aim for a healthy rate of weight loss, about 1–2 pounds per week.
- Continue taking prenatal vitamins as directed by your healthcare provider to fill any nutritional gaps.
- Curb your caffeine intake, especially if you're breastfeeding, as it can pass through breast milk and affect your baby.
- Minimize empty calories from foods high in added sugars, unhealthy fats, and sodium.
- Avoid fish high in mercury, such as shark, swordfish, king mackerel, tuna, and tilefish, as mercury can be harmful to both you and your baby.
- Avoiding alcohol is best, but according to the CDC (Centers for Disease Control and Prevention, 2024), moderate consumption is not thought to be harmful. Limit alcohol consumption to one standard drink per day and wait at least two hours before nursing.

Best Foods for Postpartum Recovery

- **Salmon:** Rich in omega-3 fatty acids, which support brain function and may help reduce the risk of postpartum depression.
- **Low-fat dairy products:** Provide calcium, protein, and vitamin D, which are essential for bone health and overall recovery.

- **Lean beef:** An excellent source of iron, which is crucial for preventing anemia and promoting healing.
- **Legumes:** Packed with fiber, protein, and various vitamins and minerals that support digestive health and overall nutrient intake.
- **Blueberries:** High in antioxidants, which help combat oxidative stress and inflammation in the body.
- **Brown rice:** A whole grain that provides complex carbohydrates, fiber, and various vitamins and minerals.
- **Oranges:** Rich in vitamin C, which aids in wound healing, collagen production, and immune function.
- **Eggs:** Provide high-quality protein, choline, and various vitamins and minerals essential for postpartum recovery.
- **Whole-wheat bread:** A good source of complex carbohydrates, fiber, and B vitamins, which help maintain energy levels and support digestive health.
- **Leafy greens:** Packed with vitamins A, C, K, and folate, which support immune function, wound healing, and overall health.
- **Whole-grain cereal:** Provides complex carbohydrates, fiber, and various vitamins and minerals to support energy levels and overall nutrient intake.

Every mother's nutritional needs are unique, so listening to your body is essential. When you make informed choices and nourish your body with a variety of healthy foods, you can support your recovery and well-being.

Hydration

Staying properly hydrated is crucial during the postpartum period, as it supports your body's healing process, maintains energy levels, and promotes milk production if you're breast-feeding. Let's explore the importance of hydration and some tips for staying adequately hydrated (Hughes, n.d.; *Keeping Hydrated During Pregnancy and the Postpartum Period*, 2022):

Importance of Hydration for Postpartum Care

Proper hydration is essential for various bodily functions, including temperature regulation, nutrient transport, and waste removal. During the postpartum period, adequate hydration is particularly important for the following reasons:

- **Supporting recovery:** Drinking enough fluids helps your body heal and recover from the physical stress of childbirth.
- **Promoting milk production:** If you're breastfeeding, staying hydrated is crucial for maintaining an adequate milk supply.
- **Preventing constipation:** Adequate fluid intake can help prevent constipation, a common postpartum issue.
- **Maintaining energy levels:** Dehydration can lead to fatigue, which is especially challenging when caring for a newborn.

Tips for Proper Hydration

- Drink water regularly throughout the day, aiming for at least 8–10 cups (64–80 ounces) of water daily. A good rule of thumb is to drink an 8-ounce glass of water every hour of the day, and a little extra if you are breastfeeding—aim for an extra 4 cups of water per day (Mehta, 2022).
- Add an electrolyte mix to at least one glass of water per day to ensure adequate water and electrolyte intake, both of which are essential to keep you hydrated.
- Monitor urine color to roughly gauge your hydration status. Clear or light-colored urine is a good indicator of adequate hydration, while dark-colored urine may signal dehydration.
- Avoid sugary or caffeinated beverages, as they can have diuretic effects and increase urine output, potentially leading to dehydration. This is why you want to avoid sugary electrolyte mixes.
- Include foods with high water content in your diet, such as fruits, vegetables, and soups, as they can contribute to overall hydration.
- Be mindful of exercise intensity and duration, as well as environmental factors like heat and humidity. Make sure that you drink at least 7–10 ounces of water every 10–20 minutes if you are exercising in really hot or humid conditions.
- Plan and prepare for hydration during workouts. It is hard to stay hydrated if you do not have a full water bottle with you. A great tip is to develop a routine. So,

for example, if you are circuit training, get into the habit of grabbing some water after each round of your circuit.

- Remember to always seek advice from your healthcare provider regarding specific hydration needs and concerns during pregnancy and postpartum, especially if you have any medical conditions or complications.

Following these tips for proper hydration can help support your body's recovery, maintain energy levels, and ensure adequate milk production if you're breastfeeding.

5-Day Meal Plan

To help you get started with your postpartum nutrition journey, I've put together a sample 5-day meal plan. This plan is designed to provide a balance of essential nutrients, support recovery, and promote overall well-being. Feel free to mix it up or experiment with your own recipes based on your preferences and dietary needs.

Day 1

- **Breakfast:** Scrambled eggs with spinach and whole-grain toast
- **Lunch:** Quinoa salad with grilled chicken, avocado, and mixed vegetables
- **Dinner:** Baked salmon with sweet potato wedges and steamed broccoli
- **Sweet treat:** Chocolate avocado pudding

Day 2

- **Breakfast:** Overnight oats with berries and nuts
- **Lunch:** Lentil soup with a side salad and whole-grain crackers
- **Dinner:** Stir-fried tofu with brown rice and mixed vegetables
- **Sweet treat:** Nut butter energy balls

Day 3

- **Breakfast:** Greek yogurt parfait with granola and fresh fruit
- **Lunch:** Turkey and hummus wrap with carrot sticks
- **Dinner:** Slow-cooker chili with lean ground beef, beans, and vegetables
- **Sweet treat:** Chia pudding with coconut milk and fresh berries

Day 4

- **Breakfast:** Whole-grain waffle with almond butter and sliced banana
- **Lunch:** Caprese salad with fresh mozzarella, tomatoes, and basil
- **Dinner:** Grilled chicken with quinoa and roasted vegetables
- **Sweet treat:** Baked apple with cinnamon and a dollop of Greek yogurt

Day 5

- **Breakfast:** Smoothie bowl with spinach, frozen berries, and protein powder
- **Lunch:** Low-mercury tuna salad with mixed greens and whole-grain bread
- **Dinner:** Vegetarian lasagna with a side salad
- **Sweet treat:** Dark chocolate-dipped strawberries

Journal Prompts

How about gifting yourself a few minutes for journaling today? To help you think about your current relationship with food and nutrition, consider taking time to reflect on the following prompts:

- How has your relationship with food changed since becoming a mother?
- What nutrients do you feel you may be lacking in your current diet?
- Describe a meal that makes you feel nourished and energized.
- How can you incorporate more fruits and vegetables into your daily routine?
- What small changes can you make to your eating habits to support your postpartum recovery?

Key Takeaways and What's Next

Throughout this chapter, we've looked into the vital role of nutrition and hydration in the postpartum period. We explored the importance of consuming a balanced diet rich in essential nutrients like protein, calcium, iron, and various vitamins to support recovery, milk production, and overall well-being. We also discussed the significance of staying adequately hydrated and provided tips for ensuring proper hydration.

Remember, nourishing your body with the right foods and fluids is crucial for your recovery and your baby's development. A healthy postpartum diet and proper hydration can help you heal, maintain energy levels, and provide the best possible nutrition for your growing baby if you are breastfeeding.

It's essential to consult with your healthcare provider for personalized guidance on postpartum nutrition and hydration needs, especially if you have any pre-existing medical conditions or complications. They can help you create a plan that meets your unique requirements and addresses any specific concerns you may have.

Don't forget that taking care of yourself is just as important as taking care of your newborn. Prioritizing your own nutrition and hydration supports your physical recovery and promotes your mental well-being. When you feel nourished and cared for, you're better equipped to handle the challenges and joys of motherhood.

In Chapter 3, we will focus on the importance of sleep during the postpartum period. We'll explore strategies for getting the rest you need, even with a newborn, and discuss how sleep plays a crucial role in your overall recovery and well-being.

THREE

Rest and Rejuvenation—Finding Peace in Postpartum Sleep

Hey Mama, I know you're tired. But I hope under that exhaustion you feel some pride, too. Because no matter how the past 24 hours went, you can fall into bed tonight knowing you made someone's life a little better today— just by loving them like only you can.

Casey Huff

The exhaustion of motherhood is intense. But do you know what? So is the immense love and pride that comes with nurturing your little one. One thing I want you to keep close in your mind while navigating this chapter and this period in your life is how nothing lasts forever. And even though the exhaustion may feel endless at times, it will pass.

Sleep during the postpartum period can be elusive, with the demands of a newborn often taking precedence over your own rest. However, prioritizing and optimizing the sleep you do get is essential for your well-being and your ability to care for your baby with the love and attention they deserve.

This chapter will explore the challenges of postpartum sleep and offer strategies to help you find moments of rest and rejuvenation amidst the beautiful chaos of new motherhood. We'll look at the importance of sleep for your physical and emotional recovery, discuss common sleep obstacles, and provide practical tips for creating a sleep-friendly environment and routine.

While the postpartum period may not allow for the uninterrupted, lengthy sleep you once enjoyed, there are ways to make the most of the rest you do get. When you understand your unique sleep needs, cultivate a supportive sleep environment, and embrace a flexible and compassionate approach, you'll discover that you can experience the restorative power of sleep, even in small doses.

The Importance of Sleep

Sleep is a crucial part of postpartum recovery, but it is often one of the most challenging aspects of new motherhood. The demands of caring for a newborn can leave you exhausted and sleep-deprived, but prioritizing rest is essential for your physical and emotional well-being.

The connection between sleep and postpartum depression is particularly significant. According to Dr. Osborne (Reed, n.d.), "There is a direct connection between lack of sleep and postpartum depression, which affects about 1 in 8 women. The two feed on each other." When you're not getting enough sleep, your risk of developing postpartum depression increases.

But this is also a double-edged sword because if you're already experiencing symptoms of depression or anxiety, falling asleep and staying asleep can become even more difficult, further impacting your emotional health. This is why it's so important to address both sleep and mental health during the postpartum period.

In addition to the increased risk of postpartum depression, sleep deprivation can lead to a host of other consequences that can make the already challenging journey of new motherhood even more difficult. Irritability is a common side effect of lack of sleep, which can strain relationships with your partner, family, and friends. When you're exhausted, your patience may wear thin, and you may find yourself snapping at loved ones or feeling easily frustrated.

Sleep deprivation can also increase the risk of accidents and injuries. When you're not well-rested, your coordination, judgment, and reaction times can be impaired, making everyday tasks like driving or handling your baby more dangerous. This is especially concerning for new mothers who may be recovering from childbirth and adjusting to the physical demands of caring for an infant.

Moreover, the emotional toll of sleep deprivation can be significant. Lack of sleep can exacerbate feelings of anxiety and depression, making it harder to cope with the challenges of motherhood. You may feel overwhelmed, hopeless, or unable to enjoy the precious moments with your baby.

Prioritizing sleep is not always easy, but it is essential for your well-being and your ability to care for your baby.

Sleep Strategies

While getting a full night's sleep may seem like an impossible dream right now, I promise you there are strategies you can implement to improve the quality and quantity of your rest.

One effective strategy is to **split up nighttime duties with your partner**. If you're breastfeeding, your partner can help by bringing the baby to you for feedings, changing diapers, or soothing the baby back to sleep. If you're bottle-feeding, take turns with the feedings to allow each other longer stretches of uninterrupted sleep.

Another important strategy is to **sleep when your baby sleeps** and go to bed when your baby does. It can be tempting to use your baby's naptime to catch up on chores or enjoy some alone time, but prioritizing sleep is crucial. Even if you can't fall asleep, quietly resting can still be restorative.

While it may be tempting to bring your baby into bed with you for convenience or comfort, it's generally not recommended to let your baby sleep with you. Co-sleeping can increase the risk of accidents and make it harder for everyone to get quality sleep.

It's also important to remember that it's okay to let your baby fuss and cry sometimes. If you've met all their needs and they're still crying, it's not harmful to let them cry for a short period while you take a few minutes to regroup.

Incorporating **relaxation techniques and meditation** into your bedtime routine can help you unwind and fall asleep more easily. Deep breathing, progressive muscle relaxation, or guided meditations can all be helpful tools.

Don't hesitate to **ask for and accept help** from family and friends. Whether it's watching the baby so you can nap or helping with household chores, accepting support can significantly improve your ability to get the rest you need.

Remember that this challenging phase is only temporary. Your baby will eventually develop more predictable sleep patterns, and you will get more rest. In the meantime, try to **avoid long naps during the day** that can interfere with nighttime sleep, **create sleep rituals** to signal to your body that it's time to wind down, and **avoid screen time before bed**, as the blue light can disrupt your natural sleep-wake cycle.

Finding what works best for you and implementing these strategies will help you prioritize your sleep so that you can get the rest and rejuvenation you need to navigate the postpartum period with greater ease and resilience.

Creating a Good Sleep Environment

Alongside all the sleep strategies mentioned above, I want to discuss creating a sleep-friendly environment and how crucial it is for promoting restful and rejuvenating sleep during this phase. Your bedroom should be a sanctuary that encourages relaxation and supports your body's natural sleep-wake cycle —this is true for everyone, but it can be really helpful when you are in the throes of new motherhood. Here are some tips to help you create the ideal sleep environment (Martinez, 2024; Suni & Rehman, 2023; Tirtadji, 2019):

- **Start by decluttering your room:** A tidy, organized space can help reduce stress and promote a sense of calm. Remove any unnecessary items, and only keep what you need for sleep and relaxation.
- **Reduce light exposure in your bedroom, especially at night:** Invest in blackout curtains or shades to block out external light and consider using a dim nightlight for nighttime feedings or diaper changes. Minimize the use of electronic devices that emit blue light, as this can interfere with your body's production of the sleep hormone melatonin.
- **Add essential oils to your sleep routine:** Using essential oils can help signal to your body that it's time to relax and unwind. Consider oils that are known for their calming properties, such as lavender, chamomile, and bergamot. Use an essential oil diffuser or sprinkle a few drops on your pillow to create a soothing, aromatic environment.
- **Consider furniture arrangement:** When arranging your bedroom furniture, emphasize symmetry and balance. A symmetrical layout can create a sense of harmony and promote relaxation. Position your bed in a way that allows for easy access to your baby's sleeping area, if necessary.
- **Find the right pillow for proper support and comfort:** Consider your sleeping position and any postpartum body changes when selecting a pillow. A

supportive pillow can help alleviate pain and promote proper alignment.

- **Look at your mattress:** If your mattress is old or unsupportive, investing in a new one can make a significant difference in your sleep quality. Look for a mattress that provides the right level of firmness and support for your body's needs.
- **Now, check your sheets:** Similarly, new sheets can contribute to a more comfortable sleep environment. Choose breathable, natural fabrics like cotton or bamboo that promote airflow and temperature regulation.
- **What about sounds?:** If you are sensitive to noise, consider using a sound machine or white noise app to create a consistent, soothing background sound. This can help mask disruptive noises and promote a more peaceful sleep environment.

These tips can help you create a more sleep-friendly environment and improve your chances of getting the rest you need. Remember, small changes can make a big difference in your sleep quality and overall well-being.

Quick Meditation for Sleep

Meditation can be really useful when it comes to getting better sleep, too. Incorporating a short meditation practice into your bedtime routine can help calm your mind, reduce stress, and promote better sleep. Here's a simple guided meditation you can try:

1. Find a comfortable position, either sitting or lying down. Close your eyes and take a few deep breaths, allowing your body to settle into stillness.

2. Begin by focusing your attention on your breath. Pay attention to the air moving in and out of your nostrils and notice the rise and fall of your chest. If your mind wanders, gently redirect your focus back to your breath.

3. Now, start to relax your body progressively. Bring your awareness to your toes and imagine them softening and releasing any tension. Slowly move your attention up through your feet, ankles, calves, knees, thighs, and hips, allowing each part of your body to relax and let go.

4. Continue moving your awareness up through your torso, back, chest, shoulders, arms, and hands. Imagine any tension or stress melting away with each exhalation.

5. Next, bring your focus to your neck, jaw, and facial muscles. Soften your jaw, relax your tongue, and release any tension in your forehead and temples.

6. Now, bring your attention back to your breath. Notice the sense of calm and relaxation that has settled over your body. Allow yourself to rest in this peaceful state, knowing that you can return to this feeling of tranquility whenever you need it.

7. When you're ready, gently open your eyes and take a moment to appreciate the sense of calm and relaxation you've cultivated.

Journaling Prompts for Better Sleep

Incorporating a journaling practice into your bedtime routine can help quiet your mind, process your emotions, and cultivate a sense of peace and relaxation that promotes better sleep. Before bedtime help your mind unwind and prepare for the rest ahead by using one of these prompts:

- What are three things you're grateful for today? Take a moment to appreciate the positive aspects of your life and cultivate a sense of gratitude before bed.
- Write about a peaceful, calming scene in nature. Engage your senses and describe the sights, sounds, smells, and sensations you imagine.
- Reflect on a challenging situation or emotion you experienced today. How can you reframe your thoughts around this experience in a more positive, compassionate light?
- What are your intentions for tomorrow? Write down a few simple, achievable goals or affirmations to help you wake up with a sense of purpose and positivity.
- Write a letter of self-compassion to yourself. Acknowledge your efforts, forgive your imperfections, and offer yourself the same kindness and understanding you would extend to a dear friend.

Key Takeaways and What's Next

We've dived into the vital role of sleep in postpartum recovery and the unique challenges new mothers face in getting the rest they need.

As a new mother, you are faced with the incredible responsibility of caring for a tiny, dependent human being, and that requires a great deal of energy and resilience. When you prioritize your own rest and rejuvenation, you are giving yourself the tools and resources you need to show up as the best version of yourself for your baby and your family.

I encourage you to try the strategies discussed in this chapter and find what works best for you and your unique situation. Whether it's incorporating a quick meditation before bed, journaling to process your thoughts and emotions, or simply giving yourself permission to rest when you can, small steps can make a big difference in your sleep quality and overall well-being.

As you move forward on your postpartum journey, remember to be patient and compassionate with yourself. Getting adequate sleep may feel like an uphill battle some days, but by consistently implementing these strategies and making rest a priority, you will begin to see improvements in your energy levels, mood, and ability to cope with the demands of motherhood.

In Chapter 4, we will focus on the role of physical activity in postpartum recovery. We'll explore the benefits of exercise for both physical and mental health, discuss safe and effective ways to incorporate movement into your daily routine, and provide practical tips for overcoming common barriers to postpartum fitness.

FOUR

Regaining Strength—Postpartum Exercise and Wellness

Postpartum is a quest back to yourself. Alone in your body again. You will never be the same. You are stronger than you were.

Amethyst Joy

The postpartum journey truly goes beyond the incredible task of bringing new life into the world; it is a time to reconnect with your body and discover a new kind of strength. While the focus is often on the physical recovery from childbirth, the postpartum period also presents an opportunity to develop a deeper sense of self and embrace the power of your own strength and resilience.

Here, we will explore the role of exercise and physical activity in postpartum recovery and well-being. We'll discuss the many benefits of incorporating safe and effective exercise routines into your postpartum journey, from regaining physical strength and stamina to enhancing mental health and emotional resilience.

For many new mothers, the idea of exercising after giving birth can feel daunting, especially when faced with the demands of caring for a newborn and the physical challenges of recovery. However, with the right approach and guidance, postpartum exercise can be an empowering tool for healing and self-discovery.

Importance of Exercise for Postpartum Care

Exercise plays a crucial role in postpartum care, offering numerous benefits for both your physical and mental well-being. Engaging in regular physical activity can help you recover from childbirth, regain strength, and promote overall health.

One of the most significant benefits of postpartum exercise is its **positive impact on mood**. Physical activity triggers the release of endorphins, the body's natural "feel-good" chemicals, which can help alleviate symptoms of postpartum depression and anxiety (Schroeder, 2024). Exercise also provides **a much-needed break** from the demands of new motherhood, allowing women to focus on their own well-being and reduce stress levels.

In addition to its mood-boosting effects, postpartum exercise **helps maintain cardiorespiratory fitness**, which may have declined during pregnancy. Engaging in aerobic activities, such as brisk walking or swimming, can improve heart health, increase endurance, and boost energy levels, making it easier to cope with the physical demands of caring for a newborn (Cleveland Clinic, n.d.).

Exercise also plays a key role in postpartum **weight management**. Many women are eager to lose the weight gained during pregnancy, and regular physical activity can help promote healthy weight loss when combined with a balanced diet. However, it's important to approach postpartum weight loss gradually and under the guidance of a healthcare provider to ensure the body has sufficient time to heal and recover.

When it comes to starting a postpartum exercise routine, the timing can vary depending on individual circumstances. Generally, gentle exercises like walking can be initiated within a few days after giving birth, or as soon as the mother feels comfortable. However, it's crucial to consult with a doctor before beginning any exercise program to ensure it's safe and appropriate for your specific situation.

For uncomplicated vaginal deliveries, most women can resume exercise around six weeks postpartum, as the majority of the physical changes that occur during pregnancy will have returned to normal. However, those who experienced a cesarean section, difficult birth, or complications may need to wait longer before engaging in physical activity. It's essential to listen to your body and gradually ease into an exercise routine, starting with simple, low-impact movements and progressively increasing intensity over time.

As a new mom, beginning an exercise program can feel really overwhelming. You can start with short 10-minute exercise sessions, as even these can provide benefits. Once you find your rhythm, increase the time you spend on this. Aim to stay active for 20–30 minutes a day, focusing on exercises that target major muscle groups, including the abdominals and back. Gradually incorporate moderate-intensity activities, such as brisk walking or swimming, and remember to always stop exercising if you experience pain or discomfort.

Low-impact activities like walking, yoga, Pilates, and gentle strength training are excellent options for postpartum exercise. Many fitness centers and community organizations offer specialized postpartum fitness classes, some of which even accommodate babies, providing a supportive environment for new mothers to exercise and connect with others in similar circumstances.

Remember, the key to a successful postpartum exercise routine is to start slowly, listen to your body, and gradually increase intensity under the guidance of your healthcare provider.

Physical Activities for Postpartum Moms

When it comes to postpartum exercise, it's essential to focus on activities that help rebuild core strength, improve pelvic floor function, and gradually increase overall fitness. Below are some of the best exercises for postpartum moms, along with guidelines on how to perform them safely and effectively (Lindberg, 2020a; Mayo Clinic Staff, 2024; Tommy's, n.d.).

Remember to always listen to your body and stop if you experience pain or discomfort. It's also crucial to consult with your healthcare provider before starting any postpartum exercise program, especially if you had a complicated delivery or underwent a cesarean section. With patience, consistency, and proper guidance, these exercises can help you safely regain strength, improve core stability, and promote overall postpartum recovery.

Pelvic Floor Exercises (Kegels)

Kegel exercises help strengthen the pelvic floor muscles, which can be weakened during pregnancy and childbirth.

1. Locate your pelvic floor muscles by imagining you're trying to stop the flow of urine.
2. Contract these muscles, hold for 5–10 seconds, then relax for 5–10 seconds.
3. Repeat 10–15 times, 3–4 times a day.

Diaphragmatic Breathing

Belly breathing helps to engage the deep abdominal muscles and promote relaxation. It works the diaphragm and transverse abdominis.

1. Lie on your back with your knees bent and feet flat on the floor.
2. Place one hand on your chest and the other on your belly.
3. Breathe deeply through your nose, allowing your belly to rise while keeping your chest relatively still.
4. Exhale slowly through pursed lips, feeling your belly fall.
5. Repeat for 5–10 breaths several times a day.

Walking

Walking is a low-impact aerobic exercise that improves cardiovascular health and promotes overall recovery.

1. Start with short, gentle walks and gradually increase distance and pace as your strength and stamina improve.
2. Aim for 10–15 minutes per day, eventually working up to 30 minutes or more.
3. Use a supportive stroller or baby carrier to bring your little one along.

Swiss Ball Bird Dog Holds

This exercise helps to improve core stability and balance while engaging the back and glute muscles.

1. Kneel on a mat with your hands resting on a Swiss ball (or a rolled-up towel if you don't have a ball), shoulders directly over your hands.
2. Engage your core and lift your right arm and left leg off the ground, extending them straight out.
3. Hold for 5–10 seconds, then return to the starting position.
4. Repeat on the opposite side, alternating for 10–15 repetitions.

Cat-Cow in Tabletop

Cat-Cow stretches help to improve spinal mobility and promote relaxation.

1. Start on your hands and knees, with your wrists under your shoulders and knees under your hips.
2. Inhale, dropping your belly and lifting your chin and tailbone toward the ceiling (Cow pose).
3. Exhale, rounding your spine, tucking your chin to your chest, and drawing your tailbone under (Cat pose).
4. Repeat for 10–15 breaths, moving slowly and smoothly between each pose.

Swiss Ball Glute Bridge

Glute bridges help to strengthen the glutes, hamstrings, and core while promoting pelvic stability.

1. Lie on your back with your feet resting on a Swiss ball (or a rolled-up towel if you don't have a ball), knees bent at a 90-degree angle.
2. Engage your core and glutes, then lift your hips off the ground until your body forms a straight line from your knees to your shoulders.
3. Hold for 5–10 seconds, then slowly lower back down.
4. Repeat for 10–15 repetitions.

Postpartum Planks (aka Standard Plank Hold)

Planks are an excellent exercise for strengthening the core, shoulders, and back.

1. Start on your hands and knees, then lower your forearms to the ground, elbows under your shoulders.

2. Step your feet back, coming into a straight line from your head to your heels.
3. Engage your core, glutes, and legs, keeping your spine neutral and your hips level.
4. Hold for 10–30 seconds, gradually increasing duration as your strength improves.

Side Plank Leg Lifts

Side plank leg lifts target the obliques, glutes, and outer thighs while improving lateral stability.

1. Lie on your side with your elbow directly under your shoulder, feet stacked.
2. Lift your hips off the ground, forming a straight line from your head to your feet.
3. Keeping your core engaged, lift your top leg a few inches, hold for 1–2 seconds, then lower.
4. Do 10–15 repetitions on each side.

Exercises for C-Section Moms

Mothers who have undergone a cesarean section (C-section) require special care and attention when it comes to postpartum exercise. It's essential to start with gentle movements that promote healing and gradually progress to more challenging exercises.

Remember to always consult with your healthcare provider before starting any exercise routine after a C-section. They can provide personalized guidance based on your individual recovery and healing process. Start slowly, listen to your body, and stop if you experience pain or discomfort. As your strength and endurance improve, you can gradually progress to more challenging exercises under the guidance of your doctor or a qualified postpartum fitness professional.

Here are some exercises specifically suited for C-section moms (Fox, 2023; Freutel, 2018):

Diaphragmatic Breathing

Refer to instructions in Diaphragmatic Breathing in the section above.

Seated Kegels

1. Sit comfortably in a chair with your feet flat on the ground.
2. Locate your pelvic floor muscles by imagining you're trying to stop the flow of urine.
3. Contract these muscles, hold for 5–10 seconds, then relax for 5–10 seconds.
4. Repeat 10–15 times, 3–4 times a day.

Wall Sit

Wall sits help to strengthen the legs and core while placing minimal stress on the incision site. These work the quadriceps, glutes, and core.

1. Stand with your back against a wall, feet shoulder-width apart and about 2 feet from the wall.
2. Slowly slide down the wall, lowering your body as if you were sitting in a chair.

3. Keep your back straight and your knees bent at a 90-degree angle.
4. Hold this position for 10–30 seconds, then slowly slide back up the wall.
5. Repeat for 3–5 repetitions.

Cesarean Delivery Scar Massage

Scar massage helps to promote healing, reduce adhesions, and improve the appearance of the scar.

1. Wait until your incision has fully healed and your doctor has given you the go-ahead to massage the area.
2. Apply a small amount of moisturizer or oil to your fingers.
3. Gently massage the scar and surrounding tissue using small, circular motions.
4. Apply light pressure, gradually increasing as your comfort level allows.
5. Massage for 5–10 minutes, 1–2 times a day.

Leg Slides

Leg slides help to gently engage the core and leg muscles without putting excessive strain on the incision site. This will work your transverse abdominis, hip flexors, and quadriceps.

1. Lie on your back with your knees bent and feet flat on the floor.
2. Engage your core by drawing your belly button toward your spine.

3. Slowly slide one foot forward, straightening your leg while keeping your back flat on the ground.
4. Slide your foot back to the starting position.
5. Repeat with the opposite leg.
6. Perform 10–15 repetitions on each side.

Simple Yoga for Postpartum Recovery

Incorporating gentle yoga practice into your postpartum routine can help promote physical and emotional healing, improve flexibility, and reduce stress. Aim to spend up to 20 minutes each day performing this simple yoga sequence, focusing on breath and body awareness (Waller, 2023). Remember to listen to your body and only move within a comfortable range.

Chair Pose

1. Stand with your feet together, then sit back as if you were sitting in a chair.
2. Raise your arms overhead, keeping your shoulders relaxed and your core engaged.
3. Hold for 5–10 breaths, then return to standing.

Child's Pose

1. Kneel on the floor with your big toes touching and your knees slightly wider than hip-width apart.
2. Sit back on your heels and fold forward, extending your arms in front of you.

3. Rest your forehead on the ground or a yoga block and breathe deeply for 5–10 breaths.

Prone Chest Stretch

1. Lie on your stomach with your hands placed under your shoulders.
2. Gently press your hands onto the floor, lifting your head and chest off the ground.
3. Keep your pelvis and legs grounded and your elbows close to your body.
4. Hold for 5–10 breaths, then lower back down.

Supported Bridge Pose

1. Lie on your back with your knees bent and feet flat on the floor, hip-width apart.
2. Place a yoga block or firm pillow under your sacrum (the triangular bone at the base of your spine).
3. Allow your arms to rest by your sides, palms facing up.
4. Hold for 5–10 breaths, then remove the block and lower your hips back to the ground.

Legs Up the Wall

1. Sit with one hip close to a wall, then swing your legs up the wall as you lie back.
2. Rest your arms by your sides, palms facing up.
3. Close your eyes and breathe deeply for 5–10 minutes.

Savasana

1. Lie on your back with your legs extended and your arms resting by your sides, palms facing up.
2. Close your eyes and focus on your breath, allowing your body to fully relax.
3. Stay in this pose for 5–10 minutes, then gently roll to your side and slowly sit up.

Journal Prompts

Journaling is a wonderful way to connect with your innermost thoughts and feelings, and it doesn't need to take long. Here are some journal prompts to help you think about your relationship with your body and your own fitness journey:

- What physical and emotional changes have you noticed in your body since giving birth, and how can you show yourself compassion during this time?
- Describe a moment when you felt proud of your body's strength and resilience during your postpartum journey.
- How has your relationship with exercise and physical activity changed since becoming a mother, and what new goals or intentions do you have for your fitness journey?
- What self-care practices, in addition to exercise, can you incorporate into your daily routine to support your overall well-being?
- Reflect on a challenging moment during your postpartum recovery and write about how you can

reframe this experience as an opportunity for growth and self-discovery.

Key Takeaways and What's Next

This chapter has explored the crucial role of exercise in postpartum recovery and overall well-being. We discussed the numerous benefits of physical activity, including improved mood, maintenance of cardiorespiratory fitness, better weight control, reduced risk of depression and anxiety, and increased energy levels.

You also found guidance on when to start exercising after giving birth, emphasizing the importance of listening to your body and consulting with your healthcare provider. Gentle exercises like walking can generally be initiated within a few days after delivery, while more intense activities should be gradually introduced around six weeks postpartum or later, depending on your individual circumstances.

Throughout the chapter, we presented a variety of exercises tailored specifically for postpartum mothers, such as pelvic floor exercises, diaphragmatic breathing, walking, and gentle strengthening moves like Swiss ball bird dog holds and glute bridges. We also included a simple yoga routine designed to promote physical and emotional healing, improve flexibility, and reduce stress.

Remember to listen to your body and start slowly. Gradually increase the intensity and duration of your workouts as you feel comfortable, and don't hesitate to modify exercises based on your individual needs. Prioritize self-care and make time for exercise, even if it's just 10 minutes a day. Every small step counts and contributes to your overall health and well-being.

In Chapter 5, we will focus on postpartum breast and vaginal care. We'll discuss common concerns, provide tips for maintaining hygiene and comfort, and offer guidance on supporting your body's recovery in these sensitive areas.

FIVE

Nurturing Breast and Vaginal Health Postpartum

Our body and its form is in continuous evolution throughout our lives; it is just more noticeable and dramatic than ever after giving birth.

Kimberly Ann Johnson

The changes our bodies undergo during pregnancy and childbirth are significant and more noticeable than anything we've noticed before. This is particularly true for the sensitive areas of the breasts and vagina, which require special care and attention in the postpartum period.

After delivering your baby, you may find yourself navigating a new landscape of physical challenges and concerns. From sore, engorged breasts to vaginal discomfort and healing, the postpartum period can be a time of great adjustment and learning. It's essential to understand that these changes are a *normal* part of the process and that with the right knowledge and care, you can support your body's recovery and maintain overall hygiene and comfort.

This chapter is dedicated to providing comprehensive guidance on caring for your breast and vaginal health after childbirth. It's important to remember that every mother's experience is unique, and there is no one-size-fits-all approach to postpartum care. I encourage you to listen to your body, trust your instincts, and seek guidance from your healthcare provider whenever necessary.

I also want to touch on an emotional component of this side of postpartum care. Many new mothers will experience feelings of vulnerability, self-consciousness, or even frustration as they adapt to the changes in their bodies. If you find yourself feeling this way, I want you to know that these feelings are valid and that practicing self-compassion and patience is just as important as the physical aspects of care we're about to discuss.

Breast Concerns and Issues

After giving birth, your breasts will undergo significant changes as they prepare to nourish your baby. As discussed in Chapter 1, these changes can include increased breast size, tenderness, and changes in the color and size of your nipples and areola. The Montgomery glands, those small bumps on the areola, may also become more noticeable. While these changes are normal, some women may experience discomfort or develop specific issues that require attention.

Common breast concerns and issues encountered postpartum include (Breast Cancer Now, n.d.; Better Health Channel, n.d.; Taylor, n.d.-b):

Blood in Breast Milk

You may notice the presence of blood in your breast milk, which can range from a pink tinge to streaks of blood. In general, this is caused by cracked or damaged nipples, rusty pipe syndrome (blood from breast ducts), intraductal papilloma, or fibrocystic changes.

It's safe to continue breastfeeding but be sure to seek medical advice to rule out any underlying causes and ensure a proper latching technique.

Nipple Thrush

A yeast infection of the nipples is characterized by persistent nipple pain, redness, and sensitivity. This is caused by the overgrowth of *Candida albicans* fungus, often due to antibiotic use, a weakened immune system, or a baby with oral thrush.

Treat both mother and baby with antifungal medications, practice good hygiene, and expose nipples to air after feeding.

Dermatitis Around the Nipple

This will appear as red, itchy, or flaky skin on or around the nipples and tends to be caused by irritation from breastfeeding, eczema, or contact dermatitis from breast pads or nipple creams.

Identify and avoid any triggers, apply a fragrance-free moisturizer, and consider using a mild topical corticosteroid under medical guidance.

Mastitis

Mastitis is an inflammation of the breast tissue, often accompanied by flu-like symptoms, redness, swelling, and pain. This is caused by blocked milk ducts, engorgement, or bacterial infection.

Continue breastfeeding or expressing milk, apply warm compresses, rest, and seek medical advice for antibiotics if necessary.

Pain While Breastfeeding

Nipple or breast pain during or after breastfeeding can be caused by improper latching, tongue-tie in the baby, engorgement, or infections like mastitis or thrush.

Ensure you and your baby have a proper latching technique, try different breastfeeding positions, apply nipple cream to soothe nipples, and seek lactation support if needed.

If you experience any persistent or concerning breast issues, consult your healthcare provider or a lactation specialist for personalized guidance. They can help you identify the underlying cause and recommend appropriate treatments to alleviate discomfort and ensure successful breastfeeding.

Breast Care

Proper breast care is essential for maintaining breast health and ensuring a comfortable breastfeeding experience. Here are some tips for breast care during the postpartum period (Murray, 2021; *Care of Your Breasts*, n.d.; *Nipple Care for Breastfeeding Mums*, n.d.):

General Breast Care

- **Practice good hygiene:** Wash your hands before handling your breasts and keep your nipples clean and dry.
- **Change breast pads often:** If you use breast pads, change them frequently to prevent moisture buildup and reduce the risk of infection.
- **Wear a supportive bra:** Choose a well-fitting, supportive bra that doesn't constrict your breasts or put pressure on your nipples.
- **Ensure proper latching:** Make sure your baby is latching correctly to prevent nipple soreness and promote efficient milk transfer.
- **Remove your baby from your breast correctly:** Break the suction by gently inserting your finger into the corner of your baby's mouth before removing it from your breast.
- **Treat sore nipples immediately:** Apply nipple cream or pure lanolin to soothe and protect sore nipples.

Breast Care When Pumping

- **Keep everything clean:** Wash your hands and ensure all pumping equipment is clean and sterilized before use.
- **Use properly fitting pump flanges:** Make sure the pump flanges (the part that goes over your nipples) fit correctly to avoid discomfort and ensure efficient milk expression.

Breast Care When Weaning

- **Consult your doctor:** If you experience engorgement or discomfort during weaning, ask your doctor about medications to help reduce inflammation and pain.
- **Avoid touching your breasts:** Minimize stimulation to your breasts, as this can trigger milk production.
- **Use cold compresses:** Place cold compresses or chilled cabbage leaves on your breasts to reduce swelling and provide relief.
- **Express milk as needed:** If your breasts become uncomfortably full, pump or hand-express just enough milk to relieve the pressure.
- **Wear breast pads:** Use breast pads to absorb any leaking milk and keep your nipples dry.
- **Choose a supportive bra:** Wear a supportive, well-fitting bra to minimize discomfort and provide gentle compression.

Remember, every mother's breastfeeding journey is unique, and not everyone finds their groove right away. It may take some time to find what works best for you and your baby—and that is okay!

Breast Self-Exam

Performing regular breast self-exams is an important aspect of breast health awareness, and it's especially crucial during the postpartum period. After giving birth, your breasts undergo significant changes as they prepare to produce milk for your baby. These changes can make it more challenging to identify potential abnormalities or concerns.

During the postpartum period, your breasts may feel more tender, swollen, or lumpy than usual. You may also experience engorgement, which is when your breasts become overly full of milk, causing discomfort and firmness. These normal postpartum changes can make it difficult to distinguish between typical breast tissue and potential issues that may require medical attention.

When you familiarize yourself with the normal look and feel of your breasts during this time, you can more easily identify any changes or abnormalities that may be cause for concern. Regular breast self-exams can help you detect issues such as:

- breast lumps or masses that feel different from the surrounding tissue
- changes in breast size, shape, or symmetry
- skin changes, such as dimpling, puckering, or redness

- nipple changes, including inversion, discharge, or scaliness

Identifying these changes early on can mean prompt medical evaluation and treatment, if necessary. This is particularly important during the postpartum period, as some conditions, such as mastitis (breast infection) or blocked milk ducts, can develop quickly and require immediate attention to prevent complications.

Furthermore, while less common, pregnancy-associated breast cancer can occur during the postpartum period. Regular breast self-exams can help detect any unusual changes that may be indicative of breast cancer, allowing for early diagnosis and treatment.

It's important to note that while breast self-exams are a valuable tool for breast health awareness, they should not replace regular clinical breast exams and mammograms, as recommended by your healthcare provider. If you notice any concerning changes or have questions about your breast health during the postpartum period, don't hesitate to reach out to your doctor for guidance and support.

By incorporating breast self-exams into your postpartum self-care routine, you can take an active role in monitoring your breast health and ensuring that any potential issues are addressed in a timely manner. This not only benefits your own well-being but also allows you to continue providing the best possible care for your baby during this special time.

Follow these steps to perform a breast self-exam (Breast-cancer.org, 2024; Mayo Clinic Staff, 2022b):

Step 1: Visual Inspection

1. Stand in front of a mirror with your shoulders straight and your arms on your hips.
2. Look for any changes in the size, shape, or color of your breasts, as well as any dimpling, puckering, or redness of the skin.
3. Check for any changes in the appearance of your nipples, such as inversion or discharge.
4. Raise your arms above your head and look for the same changes.

Step 2: Physical Examination—Lying Down

1. Lie down on your back with a pillow under your right shoulder and your right arm behind your head.
2. Using your left hand, gently feel your right breast using the pads of your fingers in a circular motion.
3. Cover the entire breast from your collarbone to the top of your abdomen and from your armpit to your cleavage.
4. Use light, medium, and firm pressure to feel all the tissue in your breast.
5. Repeat the process on your left breast using your right hand.

Step 3: Physical Examination—Standing or Sitting

1. Stand or sit upright and raise your right arm.
2. Using your left hand, gently feel your right breast

using the same circular motion and varying pressure as described in Step 2.

3. Pay special attention to the area between your breast and your armpit, as this is where many breast cancers are found.
4. Repeat the process on your left breast using your right hand.

Step 4: Nipple Check

1. Gently squeeze each nipple to check for any discharge or lumps.
2. If you notice any discharge, note the color and consistency and report it to your healthcare provider.

Tips for Effective Breast Self-Exams

- Perform breast self-exams monthly, preferably a few days after the end of your menstrual period when your breasts are less tender and swollen.
- If you are postmenopausal, choose a specific day each month to perform your self-exam.
- Be consistent in your technique and cover the entire breast area, including the armpits.
- Report any changes, lumps, or abnormalities to your healthcare provider for further evaluation.

Remember, breast self-exams are not a substitute for regular clinical breast exams and mammograms. However, they are an essential component of breast health awareness and can help you become more familiar with your breasts, making it easier to detect any changes early on.

Vaginal Concerns and Issues

After giving birth, women experience various changes in their vaginal area, which can lead to discomfort and concerns. Understanding these changes and how to address them is essential for postpartum recovery and overall well-being. Let's look at some common concerns (Britt, 2022; Levine, 2022; Mayo Clinic Staff, 2023):

- **Width of vagina:** The vagina may feel wider or looser after childbirth due to stretching during delivery. It doesn't have to stay this way; Kegel exercises will strengthen the pelvic floor muscles, improving vaginal tone.
- **Vaginal dryness:** Hormonal changes post-pregnancy can lead to vaginal dryness, making intercourse uncomfortable. Using a water-based lubricant and allowing sufficient time for arousal can help alleviate discomfort.
- **Soreness and stitches:** Vaginal soreness is common, especially if you had an episiotomy or tearing during delivery. Stitches may cause discomfort and itching as they heal. Applying ice packs, using sitz baths, and taking prescribed pain medication can provide relief.
- **Discharge:** Lochia, a postpartum vaginal discharge consisting of blood, mucus, and uterine tissue, is normal and can last for several weeks. Use pads to

manage the flow, and avoid tampons to prevent infection.

- **Bleeding:** Postpartum bleeding is heaviest in the first few days after delivery and gradually decreases. If you experience heavy bleeding, large clots, or foul-smelling discharge, contact your healthcare provider.
- **Scar tissue:** Scar tissue from perineal tearing or an episiotomy may cause pain and discomfort. Massaging the area with vitamin E oil or a specially formulated scar cream can help soften the tissue and reduce sensitivity.
- **Urinary incontinence:** Weakened pelvic floor muscles can lead to urinary leakage when coughing, sneezing, or laughing. Kegel exercises and pelvic floor physical therapy can help improve bladder control.
- **Vulvar color:** The vulva may appear swollen and darker in color due to increased blood flow during pregnancy and delivery. This change is temporary and will subside as the body recovers.

Tips to address vaginal concerns:

- Practice good hygiene by keeping the area clean and dry, wiping from front to back, and changing pads frequently.
- Perform Kegel exercises regularly to strengthen pelvic floor muscles.
- Use cold compresses or sitz baths to relieve pain and swelling.

- Wear breathable cotton underwear and loose-fitting clothing to promote air circulation.
- Avoid sexual intercourse until cleared by your healthcare provider, usually around six weeks postpartum.
- Attend postpartum check-ups to monitor healing and address any concerns.
- Seek medical advice if you experience persistent pain, heavy bleeding, or signs of infection.

Remember, postpartum recovery is a gradual process, so be patient with your body and prioritize self-care to promote healing and overall well-being.

Vaginal Care

Proper vaginal care is crucial for promoting healing, preventing infections, and maintaining overall comfort during the postpartum period. Here are some essential tips for vaginal care after giving birth (Pevzner, 2022; UnityPoint Health, n.d.; HealthLink BC, 2013):

- **Keep your perineum clean:** Always wipe from front to back to avoid introducing bacteria from the anus to the vagina.
- **Use a squirt bottle:** Fill a squirt bottle with warm water and gently rinse your perineum after using the bathroom to keep the area clean and soothe discomfort.
- **Change your pad often:** Use sanitary pads to manage postpartum bleeding and change them

frequently to keep the area dry and prevent infections. Avoid using tampons until cleared by your healthcare provider.

- **Soak in a bath:** Take warm sitz baths or shallow baths with Epsom salts to promote healing, relieve pain, and reduce swelling. Avoid using bubble baths or harsh soaps that can irritate the sensitive tissue.
- **Use pads, not tampons:** Stick to sanitary pads during the postpartum period, as tampons can introduce bacteria and increase the risk of infection.
- **Sit on a soft cushion:** Use a soft cushion or a donut-shaped pillow when sitting to relieve pressure on your perineum and promote comfort.
- **Wear comfortable clothes:** Choose loose-fitting, breathable clothing and cotton underwear to allow air circulation and prevent irritation.
- **Use an ice pack:** Apply a cold compress or ice pack wrapped in a soft cloth to the perineum to reduce swelling and numb the pain. Limit cold therapy sessions to 15–20 minutes at a time.

Additional vaginal care tips:

- I mentioned this already, but it's important, so perform Kegel exercises to strengthen pelvic floor muscles and promote healing.
- Drink plenty of water to stay hydrated and support the healing process.
- Eat a balanced diet rich in fiber to prevent constipation, which can put additional pressure on the perineum.

- Attend postpartum check-ups to monitor healing and address any concerns.

If you experience persistent pain, heavy bleeding, foul-smelling discharge, or signs of infection, such as fever or chills, contact your healthcare provider immediately.

Key Takeaways and What's Next

In this chapter, we explored the essential aspects of breast and vaginal health during the postpartum period. We discussed the various changes that occur in these areas after giving birth and the common concerns and issues that new mothers may encounter.

We emphasized the importance of proper breast care, including practicing good hygiene, wearing supportive bras, ensuring proper latching during breastfeeding, and taking care of your breasts while pumping or weaning. We also addressed common breast concerns such as blood in breast milk, nipple thrush, dermatitis, mastitis, and pain during breastfeeding, providing information on their causes and management.

Then, we looked into vaginal health concerns, such as changes in vaginal width, dryness, soreness, discharge, bleeding, scar tissue, urinary incontinence, and vulvar color changes. We provided practical tips for addressing these concerns, including maintaining good hygiene, performing Kegel exercises, using cold compresses or sitz baths, wearing comfortable clothing, and avoiding sexual intercourse until cleared by a healthcare provider.

What I want you to take away from this chapter is that understanding and addressing postpartum breast and vaginal concerns is crucial for promoting healing, preventing complications, and maintaining your overall comfort and well-being. It is essential to prioritize self-care and pay attention to any changes or discomfort in these sensitive areas.

If you encounter any persistent pain, heavy bleeding, foul-smelling discharge, or signs of infection, don't hesitate to reach out to your healthcare provider for guidance and support. They can help you navigate any issues that may arise during your postpartum recovery and ensure that you receive the appropriate care and treatment.

Remember, every woman's postpartum journey is unique, and it is important to be patient and kind to yourself as your body heals and adjusts to the demands of motherhood. Staying informed, practicing proper self-care, and seeking support when needed will help you promote a healthy and comfortable recovery.

In the next chapter, we will look at the impact of stress on new mothers and provide strategies for managing and reducing stress during the postpartum period. We will explore the various sources of stress, the potential effects on both physical and mental health, and practical techniques for promoting relaxation and self-care.

Make a Difference ~ Please Leave a Review

My mission is to bring the importance of postpartum self-care to every family. But I can only fulfill that mission by reaching parents like you.

This is where you can help! People often judge a book by its cover—and its reviews. So, on behalf of every new mom out there, please consider leaving a review.

Your words could help...

- One more mom feel less overwhelmed and isolated
- One more parent find peace during the postpartum period
- One more family gain the strength to thrive during those tough early days
- One more woman to be empowered and gain confidence in her journey
- One more dream of a balanced and fulfilling motherhood become a reality

Simply scan the QR code below to share your thoughts:

Thank you from the bottom of my heart. Now, let's dive back into more strategies and insights to support your postpartum journey!

Warmly,
Ava Wells

Part III: Emotional and Mental Well-Being

Serenity in Motherhood—Managing Stress After Birth

Being a mother is learning about strengths you didn't know you had, and dealing with fears you didn't know existed.

Nishan Panwar

Motherhood truly is a time of joy, love, and personal growth. However, it also comes with its own set of challenges and fears that can be overwhelming at times. The postpartum period, in particular, can be a time of significant stress as we navigate the demands of caring for a newborn while also recovering physically and emotionally from childbirth.

It's important to note that stress is a natural response to the many changes and responsibilities that come hand-in-hand with motherhood. From the sleepless nights and constant feedings to the pressure to be the "perfect" mother, it's all too easy to feel overwhelmed and anxious. However, it's essential to realize that you are not alone in these feelings, and there are practical strategies you can use to manage stress and find moments of calm.

In this chapter, we will explore the various sources of stress that new mothers commonly experience and the potential impact on both physical and mental well-being. We'll discuss the importance of recognizing and validating your own emotions, as well as the need for self-compassion and setting realistic expectations.

Most importantly, I'll provide you with a toolbox of practical stress management techniques that you can incorporate into your daily life. From simple breathing exercises and mindfulness practices to time management strategies and self-care rituals, these tools are designed to help you navigate the pressures of new parenthood with greater resilience and serenity.

I also want to emphasize the value of building a strong support system, whether it's leaning on family and friends, joining a mothers' group, or seeking professional help when needed. A network of understanding and encouragement can help you find the strength and resources to manage stress and prioritize your own well-being.

Postpartum Stress

Stress after having a baby can seem like a given, but what is postpartum stress syndrome? All the responsibilities that come with having a baby, keeping them happy, and adjusting to the huge shifts in your life can be a lot to handle. A certain level of stress postpartum is to be expected, but postpartum stress syndrome is an emotional state that falls between the relatively mild "baby blues" and the more severe postpartum depression (Dewar, 2022).

The Common Causes of Postpartum Stress

The postpartum period is a time of significant change and adjustment, both physically and emotionally. New mothers face a number of challenges that can contribute to their heightened stress levels. One of the most common causes of postpartum stress is **poor sleep**. The demanding feeding schedule of a newborn often leads to chronic sleep deprivation, which can take a toll on a mother's mental and physical well-being.

Additionally, many new mothers experience intense **fears and anxieties about their baby's health and well-being**. They may worry excessively about their child's development, feeding habits, or sleep patterns. These concerns can be further exacerbated if the mother's expectations and hopes for pregnancy, labor, and postpartum outcomes are not met.

Body image concerns and **worries about post-pregnancy sexuality** can also contribute to postpartum stress. Many women struggle with accepting the changes in their bodies and may feel pressure to "bounce back" to their pre-pregnancy shape quickly. Insensitive comments or lack of support from healthcare providers or partners can compound these feelings of insecurity and stress.

Feelings of isolation and loneliness are also common among new mothers, especially if they lack a strong support system. The demands of caring for a newborn can make it challenging to maintain social connections, leading to a sense of disconnection and overwhelm.

Moreover, some mothers experience **guilt over having negative thoughts** about their baby or the challenges of parenthood. They may feel ashamed or judged for not meeting societal expectations of maternal bliss, further fueling their stress levels.

Financial worries and pressures related to returning to work can also weigh heavily on new mothers. The costs associated with childcare, healthcare, and basic necessities can be disconcerting, and the prospect of balancing work and family responsibilities can feel overwhelming.

The signs and symptoms of postpartum stress are varied and can show up differently for each individual. Some common indicators include (Colino & Fabian-Weber, 2023; Mind, 2022):

- excessive worry
- changes in eating and sleeping patterns
- dizziness
- feelings of dread
- hot flashes
- irritability
- anger
- impatience
- feeling wound up
- lack of concentration

- feeling worried or tense
- a sense of isolation or loneliness

It's so important to be aware of these symptoms ahead of time and to seek support if you find yourself struggling. Ignoring or dismissing the signs of postpartum stress can lead to more severe mental health issues, such as postpartum depression or anxiety.

New mothers trying to manage postpartum stress are strongly encouraged to prioritize their self-care and seek support from loved ones and healthcare professionals. This may include practicing relaxation techniques, such as deep breathing or meditation, engaging in gentle exercise, and making time for activities that promote a sense of calm and well-being (*6 Ways to Handle Postpartum Stress*, n.d.).

Building a strong support network is also essential. Communicate openly with your partner, family members, and friends about your needs and concerns. Joining a postpartum support group or seeking the guidance of a mental health professional can also provide additional tools and resources for navigating the challenges of this time.

Experiencing postpartum stress does not make you a bad mother.

This is a common and understandable response to the huge changes and responsibilities that come with welcoming a new baby into your life. Acknowledge your feelings, seek support, and prioritize your well-being, and you will successfully navigate this challenging yet incredibly rewarding journey of motherhood.

Coping Strategies

Welcoming a new baby into your life is an incredible experience, but it can also be overwhelming and stressful. As a new parent, it's essential to prioritize your well-being and find effective strategies to manage stress. Here, we are going to look at some practical tips to help you cope with the challenges of the postpartum period.

One of the most important things you can do is to **say yes to help**. Don't be afraid to accept assistance from family, friends, or even a postpartum doula! Whether it's help with household chores, meal preparation, or childcare, having a support system can make a world of difference in reducing your stress levels. And no, you are not being a burden—when people say they want to help, they do!

Another simple but powerful strategy is to **take care of your basic needs**. Make sure to shower, get dressed, and spend some time outside each day. It sounds so basic, but fresh air and a change of scenery can work wonders for your mental well-being. Even a short walk around the block can help clear your mind and boost your energy levels.

Sleep is crucial for managing stress, but it can be elusive for new parents. Make sleep a priority whenever possible. I know everyone says this, but try to nap when your baby naps, or at least allow yourself some quiet rest time, and establish a bedtime routine that helps you unwind and relax. If you have a partner, take turns caring for the baby so that each of you can get some uninterrupted rest.

It's also important to **monitor yourself for signs of post-partum depression**. Symptoms can include persistent feelings of sadness, anxiety, or hopelessness, difficulty bonding with your baby, and thoughts of self-harm. If you experience these symptoms, don't hesitate to reach out to a healthcare provider or mental health professional for support.

Physical activity is another powerful tool for managing stress. Even if you can't commit to a full workout routine, try to incorporate some gentle movement into your day. Stretching, yoga, or a short walk can help release tension and improve your mood. Remember to listen to your body and start slowly, especially if you're recovering from childbirth.

Breathing exercises can also be incredibly effective for reducing stress and promoting relaxation. Try to take a few minutes each day to focus on deep, slow breaths. Inhale through your nose, allowing your belly to expand, and exhale slowly through your mouth. This simple practice can help calm your mind and reduce feelings of anxiety.

In the early weeks and months of parenthood, it's essential to be realistic with yourself about what you can and can't accomplish. Don't hesitate to postpone those energy-draining projects or commitments that aren't essential. Focus on taking care of yourself and your baby and let go of any unnecessary pressure or expectations.

In addition to these strategies, there are many other ways to manage postpartum stress. Some new parents find **journaling or talking to a trusted friend or therapist** helpful. Others may benefit from **joining a support group for new**

parents or trying **relaxation techniques** like meditation or progressive muscle relaxation.

Remember, every parent's journey is unique, and what works for one person may not work for another. Be patient with yourself, and don't hesitate to **experiment with different coping strategies until you find what works best for you**.

Breathing Exercises

Breathing exercises are a simple yet powerful tool for managing stress and promoting relaxation. Here are three techniques you can try (Fowler, n.d.):

Deep Breathing

1. Find a comfortable position, either sitting or lying down.
2. Place one hand on your chest and the other on your belly.
3. Inhale slowly and deeply through your nose, allowing your belly to rise as your lungs fill with air.
4. Exhale slowly through your mouth, feeling your belly fall as you release the breath.
5. Repeat for several cycles, focusing on the sensation of the breath moving in and out of your body.

Breath Focus

1. Begin by finding a quiet, comfortable space where you can sit or lie down undisturbed.

2. Close your eyes and bring your attention to your breath.

3. Notice the sensation of the air moving in and out of your nostrils or the rise and fall of your chest.

4. If your mind begins to wander, gently redirect your focus back to your breath.

5. Continue this practice for several minutes, allowing yourself to be fully present with each inhalation and exhalation.

Equal Time for Breathing In and Breathing Out

1. Start by finding a comfortable seated position.

2. Close your eyes and begin to notice your natural breathing pattern.

3. Slowly count to four as you inhale through your nose.

4. Pause briefly at the top of the inhalation.

5. Then, count to four again as you exhale slowly through your mouth.

6. Pause briefly at the bottom of the exhalation.

7. Continue this pattern, keeping your inhalations and exhalations equal in length.

8. If you find it challenging to count to four, you can begin with a shorter count and gradually increase the duration as you become more comfortable with the practice.

Remember, you aren't trying to control or change your breath but to bring a sense of awareness and mindfulness to the act of breathing. With regular practice, you may find that these techniques become a valuable tool for helping you manage stress and promote a sense of calm and well-being.

Mindfulness

Mindfulness is the practice of being present and fully engaged in the current moment without judgment or distraction. It involves paying attention to your thoughts, feelings, and sensations in a nonjudgmental way, acknowledging them without becoming overwhelmed or reactive. Mindfulness can be cultivated through various techniques, such as meditation, deep breathing, and body awareness exercises.

Practicing mindfulness can be particularly important during the postpartum period. As new mothers, we often face a range of physical, emotional, and mental challenges. When we incorporate mindfulness into daily life, we can better manage stress, anxiety, and the overwhelming emotions that come with caring for a newborn. Mindfulness can also help us cope with sleep deprivation, improve our ability to bond with our babies, and enhance our overall well-being.

Here are some tips for practicing mindfulness every day (Hoshaw, 2022; Mindful Staff, 2020; Shiraz, 2023):

- **Cultivate self-compassion:** Be kind and understanding toward yourself, acknowledging that motherhood is a challenging journey. Treat yourself with the same compassion you would extend to a dear friend.
- **Manage stress and anxiety:** When feeling overwhelmed, take a few deep breaths and focus on

the present moment. Notice your thoughts and feelings without judgment and remind yourself that these challenges are temporary.

- **Embrace the present moment:** During daily activities, such as feeding or changing your baby, bring your full attention to the task at hand. Notice the sensations, sounds, and emotions associated with each moment, allowing yourself to be fully present.
- **Cope with sleep deprivation:** When struggling with fatigue, practice mindful breathing or progressive muscle relaxation to help calm your mind and body. Remind yourself that this phase will pass and prioritize rest whenever possible.
- **Manage emotional changes:** Acknowledge and accept the wide range of emotions that come with motherhood without trying to suppress or judge them. Practice labeling your emotions, which can help you gain a sense of perspective and control.
- **Seek support:** Engage in mindful communication with your partner, family, and friends. Share your experiences and emotions openly and honestly and ask for help when needed. Consider joining a postpartum support group or seeking guidance from a therapist who specializes in mindfulness-based approaches.

Remember, whether you are new to this or already familiar with it, incorporating mindfulness into your daily life is a process, and it's essential to be patient and compassionate with yourself. Even a few minutes of mindfulness practice each day can make a significant difference in your overall well-being and ability to navigate the challenges of motherhood.

15-Minute Walking Meditation

A walking meditation is a simple yet powerful way to combine mindfulness with gentle movement. This practice can help you find moments of calm and presence, even amidst the busyness of motherhood. Here's how to perform a 15-minute walking meditation:

1. Find a quiet space where you can walk comfortably, such as a park, a quiet street, or even your backyard.
2. Begin by standing still and taking a few deep breaths. Notice the sensations of your feet on the ground and the feeling of your body standing upright.
3. Start walking at a slow, comfortable pace. Focus your attention on the physical sensations of walking, such as the feeling of your feet touching the ground, the movement of your legs, and the sway of your arms.
4. As you walk, pay attention to your breath. Notice the inhale and exhale and try to synchronize your steps with your breathing.
5. If your mind begins to wander, gently bring your attention back to the sensations of walking and breathing.
6. Continue walking mindfully for 15 minutes, maintaining a relaxed pace and an open awareness of your surroundings and bodily sensations.
7. When the 15 minutes are up, come to a gentle stop.

Take a few deep breaths and acknowledge your experience before transitioning back into your day.

Daily Check-In

Checking in with yourself every day is a simple practice that can help you stay attuned to your emotional and physical needs during the postpartum period. Here's how to check in with yourself daily:

1. Set aside a few minutes each day for your check-in. Choose a time when you will likely have a few uninterrupted minutes for your check-in such as during naptime or before bed.
2. Find a quiet, comfortable space where you can sit or lie down without distractions.
3. Close your eyes and take a few deep breaths. Bring your attention inward and notice how you're feeling physically and emotionally.
4. Ask yourself a few simple questions, such as: "How am I feeling today? What do I need right now? What's bringing me joy or stress?"
5. Listen to your responses without judgment. Acknowledge your feelings and needs and consider what small steps you can take to support yourself.
6. End your check-in with a few deep breaths and a moment of self-compassion. Remind yourself that you're doing the best you can and that it's okay to prioritize your own well-being.

Journal Prompts

The following prompts will help you consider how stress is impacting your life right now. Remember that you can always return to each journal entry and reflect on how your journey is changing each day and how much you have already overcome!

- What are the main sources of stress in your life right now, and how are they impacting your well-being?
- Describe a time when you successfully managed a stressful situation. What strategies did you use, and how did you feel afterward?
- Imagine your ideal self-care routine. What activities or practices would you include, and how would they help you manage stress?
- Reflect on the role of mindfulness in your life. How can being present and aware help you navigate stressful experiences?
- Write a letter of compassion and understanding to yourself, acknowledging the challenges you're facing and offering words of support and encouragement.

Key Takeaways and What's Next

Here, we have covered postpartum stress and its impact on us as new mothers. We discussed the common causes of stress during the postpartum period, such as poor sleep, fears about the baby's health, unmet expectations, body image concerns, lack of support, and financial worries. We also examined the signs and symptoms of postpartum stress, including excessive worry, changes in eating and sleeping patterns, feelings of isolation, and physical symptoms like dizziness and hot flashes.

Taking care of your mental health as a mother is essential. Recognizing and addressing postpartum stress is crucial for your well-being and your ability to care for your baby. It's important to remember that experiencing stress during this time is normal and does not make you a bad mother.

If you find yourself feeling overwhelmed, anxious, or stressed, know that you are not alone. Many new mothers experience similar challenges, and it's okay to ask for help.

Throughout this chapter, we also discussed various coping strategies to help manage postpartum stress. These include accepting help from others, prioritizing self-care activities like showering and getting dressed, making sleep a priority, engaging in physical activity, practicing breathing exercises, and postponing energy-draining projects. Remember that finding the strategies that work best for you may take some trial and error, and that's okay.

It's also crucial to monitor yourself for signs of postpartum depression, which is a more severe condition that requires professional attention. If you experience persistent feelings of sadness, hopelessness, or difficulty bonding with your baby, don't hesitate to reach out for support.

As we move forward, Chapter 7 will explore postpartum depression in greater depth. We'll explore the signs, symptoms, and risk factors associated with this condition, as well as strategies for seeking help and support. Remember, you are not alone in this journey, and there are resources available to help you navigate the challenges of motherhood.

Take a moment to reflect on the information we have covered in this chapter and consider how you can prioritize your mental health during the postpartum period. Whether it's practicing a few minutes of deep breathing each day, reaching out to a friend for support, or scheduling an appointment with a therapist, small steps can make a big difference in managing stress and promoting your all-important personal well-being.

SEVEN

Beyond the Blues – Understanding Postpartum Depression

Postpartum depression makes you suddenly feel like a stranger to yourself, but knowing the clinical facts are the first step toward wellness.

Judy Dippel

We touched on this in the previous chapter; postpartum depression (PPD) is a common and serious mental health condition that affects many new mothers, yet it remains shrouded in stigma and misunderstanding. PPD really can make you feel like a stranger to yourself, disconnected from the joy and bond you were expecting to feel with your new baby. This sense of isolation and confusion can be overwhelming and disorienting, but understanding the clinical facts about PPD is the first step toward recognizing and overcoming this challenge.

In this chapter, I will shed some light on postpartum depression, offering insights, support, and resources for any mothers facing this difficult experience. It's important to remember that PPD is not a character flaw or a sign of weakness. It is a real and *treatable* medical condition that affects up to 1 in 7 mothers (Mughal et al., 2022). With the right support and treatment, including therapy and medication, many women are able to manage their symptoms and really embrace the joys of motherhood.

If you're currently struggling with PPD, know that you are not to blame, and that recovery is possible. You are here, arming yourself with knowledge and seeking the support you need, so I know you can begin the path toward healing and reclaiming your sense of self. Whether you're a mother, a partner, or a family member, this chapter is designed to help you better understand and support those affected by postpartum depression.

What Is Postpartum Depression?

As you know by now, PPD is a serious mental health condition that affects many new mothers after giving birth. You may even recognize this in yourself or your loved ones already. It is characterized by persistent feelings of sadness, hopelessness, and inadequacy that can interfere with a mother's ability to care for herself and her baby. PPD is more severe and long-lasting than the "baby blues," which are common feelings of worry, unhappiness, and fatigue that many women experience in the first few weeks after childbirth.

Several factors can contribute to the development of PPD, including:

- previous postpartum depression or depression not related to pregnancy
- severe premenstrual syndrome (PMS)
- a difficult or stressful marriage or relationship
- lack of support from family members or friends
- stressful life events during pregnancy or after childbirth, such as severe illness, premature birth, or a difficult delivery

Hormonal changes, sleep deprivation, and the overwhelming responsibility of caring for a newborn can also play a role in the onset of PPD.

Signs and symptoms of postpartum depression can be divided into three categories (Mayo Clinic Staff, 2022c; March of Dimes, n.d.-a):

Changes in Feelings

- You may feel depressed, like having a heavy weight on your chest that stays with you all day, every day. It's like a big dark cloud that's always there. You might feel alone, sad, or hopeless.
- Experiencing shame, guilt, or feeling like you've failed can be another sign. You might feel like you're not good enough or like you're a bad parent.
- Feeling panicked or worried a lot can be scary, but also an indication of PPD. Your heart might race, and you might find it hard to catch your breath.

- You may experience severe mood swings where your emotions can change from one extreme to another quickly. You might feel happy one moment and then very sad the next.

Changes in Everyday Life

- Losing interest in activities you normally enjoy can be a sign of PPD. Life might feel dull and uninspiring.
- Another sign is feeling tired all the time, which can be physically and mentally draining.
- PPD can bring significant changes in appetite, resulting in eating much more or less than usual, and can impact your overall well-being.
- Unintended weight gain or loss can be another concerning sign.
- You might also experience trouble sleeping or sleeping too much, which can disrupt your daily routine and mood.
- Difficulty concentrating or making decisions might also be noticed.

Changes in Thoughts About Yourself or Your Baby

- You might find it hard to connect with your baby.
- Experiencing thoughts about harming yourself or your baby can be a very distressing sign of PPD.
- You might also be having thoughts of suicide.

It's essential for new mothers and their loved ones to be aware of these signs and symptoms, as early recognition and treatment can significantly improve outcomes. If you or someone you know is experiencing symptoms of postpartum depression, it's crucial to seek help from a healthcare provider. With proper support and treatment, mothers can overcome PPD and get back to enjoying motherhood.

Baby Blues vs. PPD

Many new mothers will experience a range of different emotions after giving birth, including feelings of sadness, mood swings, and irritability. While these feelings are often referred to as the "baby blues," it's important to understand the difference between this common experience and the more severe condition of PPD.

Baby blues is a mild, short-term condition that affects up to 80% of new mothers (*Depression in Pregnant Women and Mothers*, 2004). It typically begins within a few days of giving birth and resolves on its own within a couple of weeks. The signs and symptoms of baby blues may include:

- mood changes
- impatience
- feeling like "I'm not myself today"
- crying for no apparent reason
- sadness

These feelings are often attributed to the hormonal changes that occur after childbirth, as well as the overwhelming responsibility of caring for a newborn.

In contrast, postpartum depression is a more severe and long-lasting condition that affects approximately 10–15% of new mothers (Anokye et al., 2018). PPD symptoms are more intense and can interfere with a mother's ability to care for herself and her baby. Key differences between baby blues and PPD include:

- **Duration:** Baby blues typically last for a few days to a couple of weeks, while PPD symptoms persist for longer periods, often several weeks or months.
- **Severity:** The symptoms of PPD are more severe and can significantly impact a mother's daily functioning, whereas baby blues symptoms are milder and do not typically interfere with daily life.
- **Impact on bonding:** Mothers with PPD may have difficulty bonding with their babies, while those with baby blues usually do not experience this issue.
- **Thoughts of self-harm:** Women with PPD may have thoughts of harming themselves or their babies, which is not a symptom of baby blues.

While baby blues is a common and temporary experience, PPD requires professional attention and treatment. If symptoms persist beyond a few weeks or interfere with daily functioning, it's essential to seek help from a healthcare provider.

Remember, both baby blues and PPD are *treatable* conditions, and seeking help is a sign of strength, not weakness. With proper support and care, mothers can overcome these challenges and enjoy the joys of motherhood.

Dealing With Guilt

Guilt is a common emotion experienced by new mothers, and it can be particularly intense for those struggling with PPD. "Mom guilt" refers to the feeling of not being good enough or not meeting the expectations of what a mother should be. This guilt can stem from various sources and can significantly impact a mother's mental health.

Some common reasons for mom guilt include (Zamosky, n.d.):

- not breastfeeding, not breastfeeding long enough, or not enjoying every moment of breastfeeding
- reaching out for help, feeling like they should be able to handle everything on their own
- having a bad day and not feeling like they are being the best mother they can be
- taking time for themselves, believing that they should be solely focused on their baby

These feelings of guilt can be exacerbated by societal pressures, social media, and the idealized image of motherhood often portrayed in popular culture.

For mothers with PPD, guilt can play a significant role in the severity and duration of their symptoms. Women with PPD may feel guilty for not being able to bond with their baby, for having negative thoughts about motherhood, or for not living up to their own expectations of what a mother should be. This guilt can lead to feelings of shame, worthlessness, and a reluctance to seek help.

It's important for mothers to understand that **guilt is a *normal* emotion, but it should not be allowed to control their lives or prevent them from seeking support.** Some strategies for dealing with mom guilt include (Kripke, n.d.):

- challenging negative thoughts and replacing them with more realistic, compassionate ones
- talking to other mothers and realizing that many share similar feelings and experiences
- seeking professional help, such as therapy or support groups, to work through feelings of guilt and shame
- practicing self-care and acknowledging that taking care of oneself is essential for being a good mother
- letting go of the idea of perfection and embracing the reality that all mothers have challenges and make mistakes

Experiencing guilt does not make you a bad mother. It's a common and understandable emotion, especially when dealing with PPD.

Prevention Strategies

There are strategies that can help reduce the risk or severity of this condition. Understanding the risk factors and taking proactive steps to promote mental health can make a significant difference in a new mother's postpartum experience.

Risk factors for PPD include (Familydoctor.org editorial staff, 2017; Waits, 2023):

- diagnoses of depression during pregnancy (perinatal depression)
- history of depression or other mood disorders, like bipolar disorder
- family history of postpartum depression
- difficulty breastfeeding
- experiencing abuse during pregnancy or a history of abuse
- high stress and childcare stress
- hesitancy about motherhood
- lack of social support
- dissatisfaction with your partner
- income level and confidence in your ability to take care of your baby
- traumatic birth or labor that didn't go according to plan

By educating yourself about PPD, you can learn more about its symptoms and be prepared to deal with them. Being aware of how it may affect you is the first step toward getting help when needed.

Inform your partner and family members about PPD so they can understand what you're going through. This way, they can provide the necessary support and care during this challenging time, which can make a significant difference in how you cope with the condition.

Having a plan in place for the postpartum period can be helpful, too. Assigning tasks to family members or friends can reduce your workload and prevent you from feeling overwhelmed. Accepting help and sharing responsibilities can make the transition smoother.

Identify friends who you can rely on for emotional support and practical assistance. Spending time with supportive friends can help lift your mood and make you feel less isolated during this sensitive time.

Make time for activities you enjoy, even if it's just for a short while each day. Engaging in hobbies or interests that bring you joy can help maintain your mental well-being and provide a sense of normalcy.

As we have learned, eating a balanced diet and staying physically active are essential for your overall health. Good nutrition and regular exercise can boost your mood and reduce stress levels, contributing to a more positive outlook on life.

Spending time outdoors and getting fresh air and sunlight can have a positive impact on your mental health. Being in nature can help you relax, rejuvenate, and appreciate the beauty of the world around you.

Other preventive measures include attending prenatal classes, building a strong support network, and practicing stress-reduction techniques like meditation or deep breathing exercises. If you have a history of depression or other risk factors, consider discussing your concerns with your healthcare provider early on. They may recommend additional support or treatment options to help prevent or manage PPD.

Seeking Professional Help

Seeking professional help is crucial for mothers experiencing PPD. As we have learned, PPD is a serious mental health condition that requires proper diagnosis and treatment to ensure the well-being of both the mother and the baby.

Healthcare professionals, such as obstetricians, pediatricians, or mental health specialists, can diagnose PPD through a combination of physical exams, lab tests, and psychological evaluations. They may ask questions about the mother's symptoms, feelings, and daily functioning to determine the severity of the condition.

It's essential to seek professional help when (Office on Women's Health, 2023):

- The baby blues symptoms don't go away after two weeks or are very intense.
- Symptoms of depression begin within one year of delivery and last more than two weeks.
- It is difficult to work or get things done at home.
- The mother cannot care for herself or her baby (e.g., eating, sleeping, bathing).
- The mother has thoughts about hurting herself or her baby.

Treatment options for PPD include (Mayo Clinic Staff, 2022d; WebMD Editorial Contributors, n.d.):

- **Cognitive behavioral therapy (CBT):** A type of talk therapy that helps individuals identify and change negative thought patterns and behaviors.
- **Interpersonal therapy (IPT):** A form of therapy that focuses on improving communication skills and relationships to reduce stress and improve mood.
- **Talking therapy:** A general term for any type of therapy that involves talking with a mental health professional to work through challenges and develop coping strategies.
- **Antidepressants:** Medications that help balance brain chemicals to improve mood and reduce symptoms of depression. However, it's important to note that caution should be exercised when taking antidepressants, especially for breastfeeding mothers. Some antidepressants can pass through breast milk and may have potential side effects for the baby. It's crucial to discuss the risks and benefits of antidepressants with a healthcare provider to make an informed decision.

In addition to these treatments, support groups and lifestyle changes, such as **regular exercise**, a **balanced diet**, and **sufficient rest**, can also help manage PPD symptoms.

It's important to remember that it is a positive thing to seek professional help. PPD is a treatable condition, and with the right support and interventions, mothers can recover and experience the joys of motherhood. If you or someone you know is experiencing symptoms of PPD, don't hesitate to reach out to a healthcare provider or mental health professional for guidance and support.

Journal Prompts

Journaling can help you connect deeply with your feelings. Consider the following prompts regarding the many transformations of motherhood:

- What has been the most challenging aspect of postpartum life for you, and how have you coped with it so far?
- Describe a moment of joy or connection you've experienced with your baby, no matter how small. What made that moment special?
- What are three things you're grateful for today? Spend some time appreciating the good in your life despite the challenges.
- Write a letter of encouragement to yourself, as if you were writing to a dear friend going through a similar postpartum experience. What words of support and wisdom would you offer?
- Reflect on your support system. Who are the people you can turn to for help and understanding during this time? How can you reach out and ask for the support you need?

Key Takeaways and What's Next

Here, we've looked at the important topic of PPD, a serious mental health condition that affects many new mothers. We discussed the signs and symptoms of PPD, which can include persistent feelings of sadness, guilt, or hopelessness, difficulty bonding with your baby, and changes in appetite or sleep patterns.

PPD is a real and treatable condition that requires professional support and intervention. It is not a reflection of your worth as a mother or a sign of weakness. Seeking help when needed is a brave and essential step in your postpartum journey.

We explored the various risk factors for PPD, such as a history of depression, lack of support, and stressful life events. Understanding these risk factors can help you take proactive steps to protect your mental health and build a strong support system.

Throughout the chapter, we emphasized the importance of self-care and mindfulness practices in managing PPD symptoms. Prioritizing activities that bring you joy, practicing self-compassion, and staying present in the moment can all contribute to improved mental well-being.

It's crucial to remember that every mother's journey is unique, and it's okay not to feel like you have everything under control all the time. Postpartum life is full of challenges and adjustments for every new mother, and it's normal to experience a wide range of emotions. Be gentle with yourself and remember that you're doing the best you can—and that is enough!

If you're struggling with PPD, know that you're not alone and that help is available. Don't hesitate to reach out to your healthcare provider, a mental health professional, or a supportive loved one. With the right treatment and support, you can navigate this difficult time and find joy in your motherhood journey.

In the upcoming chapter, we will focus on the important topics of body image and self-confidence during the postpartum period. We'll explore how the physical and emotional changes of pregnancy and childbirth can impact the way you see yourself and discuss strategies for cultivating a positive body image and self-love.

Remember, taking care of your mental health is just as important as caring for your physical health and your baby.

EIGHT

Body Image and Self-Confidence in Motherhood

Feeling beautiful has nothing to do with what you look like.

Emma Watson

We live in a society that often places undue pressure on women to adhere to unrealistic beauty standards, so it's essential to remember that true beauty comes from within. As new mothers, we are navigating the physical and emotional changes brought about by pregnancy and childbirth, so it is crucial that we develop a sense of self-love and appreciation for the incredible feat our bodies have accomplished.

The postpartum period can be a time of significant vulnerability and self-doubt as women adjust to their new roles and the changes in their bodies. Stretch marks, loose skin, and changes in weight and shape are all natural and common experiences, yet societal messages often frame these changes as flaws to be fixed or hidden. This pervasive narrative can lead to feelings of shame, inadequacy, and a negative body image.

However, it's time to challenge these harmful societal standards and embrace a more inclusive and empowering vision of beauty. Every mother's journey is unique, and every body tells a story of strength, resilience, and the miraculous ability to create and sustain life. By shifting our focus from external appearances to the inner qualities that make us truly beautiful, such as compassion, kindness, and the fierce love we have for our children, we can begin to cultivate a more positive and accepting relationship with our postpartum bodies.

It's important to remember that the journey to self-love and body positivity is not always linear. There may be days when negative self-talk or comparison to others creeps in, but by committing to a practice of self-compassion and gratitude, we can gradually transform our relationship with our bodies and ourselves.

Throughout this chapter, I encourage you to challenge the notion that beauty is confined to a narrow set of physical characteristics. Try to embrace the idea that true beauty radiates from within and that the love, care, and dedication you show to your child and to yourself are the most beautiful qualities of all.

Body Image and Giving Birth

The journey of pregnancy and childbirth is a life-changing experience that brings about significant physical and emotional changes. While the arrival of a new baby is a joyous occasion, the impact of these changes on a woman's body image can be huge. Many women find themselves grappling with mixed emotions as they adjust to their postpartum bodies, and societal pressures can exacerbate their feelings of self-doubt and dissatisfaction.

During pregnancy, a woman's body undergoes a series of remarkable changes to accommodate the growing life within. While some women embrace these changes and celebrate the incredible capabilities of their bodies, others may struggle with body dissatisfaction. Research has shown that body dissatisfaction during pregnancy can have serious implications for both maternal and fetal health (Salzer et al., 2023). Women who experience high levels of body dissatisfaction may resort to unhealthy behaviors, such as severely restricting their eating or engaging in excessive exercise, in an attempt to control their changing shape. For those with a history of eating disorders, pregnancy can trigger a relapse, putting both mother and baby at risk.

The postpartum period brings its own set of challenges when it comes to body image. The physical aftermath of childbirth, such as stretch marks, loose skin, and changes in breast shape and size, can be difficult to accept. Society's unrealistic expectations of "bouncing back" and achieving a pre-pregnancy body add to the pressure new mothers face. The constant images of celebrities and influencers who seem to effortlessly shed their pregnancy weight can leave many women feeling inadequate and discouraged.

It's important to recognize that negative body image can have serious consequences for mental health. Studies have shown that women who experience body dissatisfaction during the perinatal period are four times more likely to develop perinatal depression (Horsager-Boehrer, 2022). The constant self-criticism and comparison to unattainable standards can take a toll on a woman's emotional well-being, making it harder to enjoy the joys of motherhood.

However, it's crucial to remember that the changes a woman's body undergoes during pregnancy and childbirth are not flaws to be fixed but rather a testament to the incredible strength and resilience of the female body. Embracing self-compassion and gratitude for the miraculous journey of bringing new life into the world can be a powerful antidote to negative body image.

If you can shift the focus from external appearances to the incredible functions and capabilities of your body, you can cultivate a more positive and accepting relationship with your postpartum self. Surrounding yourself with supportive and uplifting influences, whether it be through social media, friends, or family, can also help foster a more positive body image.

Building a Positive Body Image

Building a positive body image is an essential aspect of self-care and well-being, especially during the journey of motherhood. Yes, societal pressures and unrealistic beauty standards can make this challenging, but there are several steps you can take to foster a more accepting and loving relationship with your body.

First and foremost, it's crucial to **accept yourself as you are**. Really embrace the unique features and characteristics that make you who you are and recognize that your worth is not defined by your physical appearance. Remember that everybody is different, and there is no one "ideal" shape or size.

When confronted with negative messages about body image, consider the source. Much of the media we consume presents a narrow and often unrealistic view of beauty. By questioning these messages and seeking out more diverse and inclusive representations, you can start to **challenge the notion that there is only one way to be beautiful**.

Developing a **positive attitude and self-talk** is another key aspect of building a healthy body image. When negative thoughts arise, try to counter them with affirmations and reminders of your body's strengths and capabilities. Surround yourself with positivity, whether through uplifting social media accounts, supportive friends and family, or inspiring quotes and mantras—having quotes up around my house has really helped me to work on my positive self-talk over the years.

As a mother, it's especially important to remember your motivation for taking care of yourself. Your body has done something miraculous in bringing new life into the world, and it deserves to be nourished and cared for with kindness and respect. Focus on building **healthy habits** that make you feel good rather than striving for an arbitrary number on the scale.

It's also essential to recognize that your body does not need to change in order to be worthy of love and acceptance. **No matter your size or shape, you deserve love and respect.** Surround yourself with people who affirm and support you and set boundaries with those who engage in body-shaming or negative talk.

Practicing **gratitude for your body** and all that it does for you can be a powerful tool in fostering a positive body image. Try to take a moment each day to appreciate the incredible functions and capabilities of your body, from your heart that beats tirelessly to the arms that hold and comfort your child.

When setting goals for yourself, **focus on health and well-being** rather than striving for a specific body type. Engage in physical activities that bring you joy and make you feel strong and capable rather than punishing yourself with grueling workouts. Nourish your body with wholesome, nutritious foods that fuel your energy and vitality.

Finally, remember to **be patient and kind to yourself.** Building a positive body image is a journey, and there will be ups and downs along the way. Celebrate your victories, no matter how small, and forgive yourself when negative thoughts or self-doubt creep in.

By taking these steps and surrounding yourself with support and positivity, you can create a more loving and accepting relationship with your body. Remember, you are worthy of self-love and respect, just as you are, and your body is a testament to your strength and resilience as a mother.

Building Self-Confidence

As a new mother, it's really common to experience moments of self-doubt and uncertainty—we all do! The challenges of caring for a newborn, coupled with the physical and emotional changes of the postpartum period, can take a toll on your self-confidence. However, by implementing some simple strategies, you can boost your self-esteem and feel more self-assured in your role as a mother.

One of the most effective ways to build self-confidence is to **start each day with intention**. Take a few moments to get ready for the day, even if it's just changing out of your pajamas and brushing your hair. This simple act of self-care can help you feel more put-together and prepared to tackle the day ahead.

Engaging in **regular exercise** is another powerful way to boost self-confidence. Physical activity releases endorphins, which can improve your mood and reduce stress (Mayo Clinic Staff, 2022a). Even a short walk or a gentle yoga session can help you feel more energized and self-assured.

Setting small, achievable goals for yourself can also help build self-confidence. Whether it's tackling a household task, learning a new skill related to parenting, or carving out time for a hobby you enjoy, accomplishing these goals can give you a sense of pride and achievement.

It's also important to make an effort to **get out of the house and connect with others**. Joining a new mom's group, attending a baby class, or simply meeting up with friends can provide a much-needed sense of community and support. Surrounding yourself with positive, encouraging people can help you feel more confident in your abilities as a mother.

Taking time for yourself is another essential aspect of building self-confidence. While it may feel selfish to prioritize your own needs, remember that self-care is not a luxury but a necessity. Whether it's taking a relaxing bath, reading a book, or pursuing a creative outlet, making time for activities that bring you joy and fulfillment can help you feel more centered and self-assured.

Working on a **positive mindset** is also crucial for building self-confidence. Pay attention to your self-talk and try to reframe negative thoughts into more supportive and encouraging ones. Surround yourself with affirmations and reminders of your strengths and capabilities.

Recognizing your unique skills and talents can also help boost your self-confidence. Take a moment to reflect on the things you're good at, whether it's your ability to soothe your baby, your creativity in coming up with new play ideas, or your knack for organization. Celebrate these strengths and let them be a source of pride and self-assurance.

It can also be really useful to **identify the people, activities, and experiences that make you feel confident and empowered** and make an effort to incorporate them into your life. Whether it's spending time with a supportive friend, engaging in a favorite hobby, or setting aside time for self-reflection, prioritizing these confidence builders can help you feel more self-assured.

Finally, remember that building self-confidence is an ongoing process. Embrace opportunities to learn and grow, both as a mother and as an individual—you could attend a parenting workshop, read books and articles that resonate with you, or seek out role models who inspire you. All of these things will help you develop a strong sense of self-confidence that will serve you well on your motherhood journey.

Affirmations

Positive affirmations can be a powerful tool in working on your self-love and body acceptance during the postpartum period. Here are some postpartum affirmations you can adopt in your life to inspire and empower you:

- My body is strong, capable, and worthy of love and respect.
- I embrace and celebrate the changes in my body as a testament to the miracle of life.
- I am more than just a body; I am a whole, complex, and beautiful person.
- I choose to nourish my body with kindness, compassion, and care.
- I am grateful for all that my body has done and continues to do for me and my baby.
- I trust my body's wisdom and its ability to heal and recover.

- I am proud of my body for its incredible strength and resilience.
- I commit to resting and recharging whenever I need it.
- I surround myself with positivity and let go of any negativity directed toward my body.
- I am at peace with my postpartum journey and trust the process.
- I find joy in movement and physical activities that make me feel good.
- I honor my body's needs and listen to its messages with compassion.
- I am grateful for the opportunity to experience the life-changing journey of motherhood.
- I choose to focus on the love and connection I share with my baby rather than my physical appearance.
- I am beautiful, inside and out, just as I am.
- I celebrate my body's unique shape and size, knowing that everybody is different and worthy of acceptance.
- I am patient and gentle with myself as I navigate the challenges of the postpartum period.
- I eat wholesome, nutrient-rich foods that support my well-being and nourish my body.
- I am confident in my ability to make healthy choices for myself and my baby.
- I find strength in the love and support of my family and friends.
- I let go of comparison and embrace my own unique postpartum journey.
- I am proud of my body for its incredible ability to create, nurture, and sustain life.

- I treat my body with the same kindness and respect that I show to my loved ones.
- I am grateful for the opportunity to model self-love and body acceptance for my child.
- I trust that I am doing my best, and that is always enough.
- I make time for activities that bring me joy and relaxation because I deserve self-care.
- I honor the wisdom and strength of all the mothers who have come before me.
- I am grateful for my body's remarkable ability to adapt and heal.
- I embrace my postpartum body as a symbol of the powerful journey of motherhood.
- I am confident in my ability to nurture and care for my baby, just as I nurture and care for myself.
- I choose to focus on the love and connection I share with my baby rather than societal expectations.
- I am grateful for the opportunity to experience the profound love and joy of being a mother.
- I trust in my body's natural ability to find its own unique balance and rhythm.
- I am worthy of self-love, self-care, and self-acceptance, always.
- I choose to embrace my postpartum journey with curiosity, compassion, and gratitude.

Creating Your Own Affirmations

If you want to work on creating your own personal affirmations, follow these simple steps:

1. Identify the negative thoughts or beliefs you wish to overcome, such as "I hate my postpartum body" or "I will never feel confident again."

2. Write down the opposite of these negative statements, focusing on what you want to feel or believe instead. For example, "I am learning to love and accept my postpartum body" or "I am growing more confident each day."

3. Refine your affirmations to make them concise, specific, and easy to remember using the present tense. Be sure to phrase them as if they are already true.

4. Repeat your affirmations daily; this can be either out loud or silently to yourself. You can say them in the mirror, write them down in a journal, or post them in a visible location as a reminder.

5. Embrace the power of repetition and consistency. The more you practice your affirmations, the more they will begin to feel true and resonate with you on a deeper level.

Affirmations are a tool for shifting your mindset and cultivating a more positive and loving relationship with yourself. It's important to be patient and compassionate with yourself as you incorporate this practice into your self-care routine.

Journal Prompts

How will you take care of yourself today? Consider grabbing your journal for some self-reflection time using the following prompts:

- Write a letter of love and appreciation to your body, thanking it for all it has done and continues to do for you.
- Reflect on a time when you felt truly confident and at peace with your body. What was different about that moment, and how can you cultivate more of that feeling in your life now?
- Imagine you are having a conversation with your younger self about body image. What wisdom and advice would you share with her?
- Make a list of your top five favorite physical features and write about why you appreciate each one.
- Reflect on the qualities and attributes you most admire in yourself beyond physical appearance. How can you nurture and celebrate these aspects of yourself more fully?

Key Takeaways and What's Next

This chapter has looked at the complex and often challenging relationship between body image and self-confidence in the postpartum period. We've discussed how the physical changes of pregnancy and childbirth can impact a woman's perception of her body and how societal pressures and unrealistic beauty standards can exacerbate feelings of self-doubt and dissatisfaction.

Most importantly, we've learned that cultivating a positive body image and self-confidence is a vital aspect of postpartum self-care and well-being. It's important to remember that the journey to self-love and body acceptance is a process, and it's okay to have moments of struggle or self-doubt along the way. What matters most is that you continue to practice self-compassion, patience, and kindness toward yourself. Surround yourself with supportive and uplifting influences, and remember that you deserve love and respect, regardless of your size or shape.

As you move forward on your postpartum journey, I encourage you to continue prioritizing self-care and self-love. Engage in activities that make you feel good, both physically and emotionally. Seek out resources and support that resonate with you, whether it be through books, online communities, or trusted friends and family members. Remember, you are not alone in this journey, and there is a wealth of support and encouragement available to you.

Most importantly, always remember that you are beautiful, worthy, and deserving of love and acceptance, just as you are. Your body has done and continues to do amazing things, and that is something to celebrate and honor. Embrace your unique journey, and know that by modeling self-love and body positivity, you are not only nurturing your own well-being but also setting a powerful example for your child.

As we move into Chapter 9, we'll be shifting our focus to the incredible bond between mother and baby. We'll explore ways to nurture and strengthen this connection, as well as strategies for overcoming common challenges and concerns.

Part IV: Bonding With Baby

NINE

Gentle Beginnings—Essentials of Newborn Bonding

All those clichés, those things you hear about having a baby and motherhood—all of them are true. And all of them are the most beautiful things you will ever experience.

Penélope Cruz

N ewborn care is a fundamental component of motherhood, and yes, it may seem daunting at times, but it is also a deeply rewarding experience. From the first time you hold your baby in your arms to the countless tender moments of nurturing and care, each of these moments strengthens the bond between mother and child. This chapter is going to give you guidance on newborn bonding, equipping you with the tools and understanding necessary to care for your baby effectively and with confidence.

Learning how to properly care for and connect with your newborn is not only essential for your baby's well-being but also a crucial aspect of your own self-care as a mother. When you feel prepared and confident in your ability to meet your baby's needs, you spend more time enjoying motherhood and developing a deeper sense of self-assurance in your role as a parent. With the knowledge and tools provided in this chapter, you can approach newborn care with confidence, fostering a deep, unbreakable bond with your child that will last a lifetime.

Newborn Behavior and Needs

Understanding your newborn's behavior is the key to providing the best possible care and fostering a strong bond with your baby. Newborns may not be able to tell you what they are feeling and what they need with words yet, but they do communicate through various cues and body language, which can help you identify their needs and respond accordingly.

You can learn to recognize and interpret your baby's cues, which will help you meet their needs more effectively—whether they are hungry, tired, uncomfortable, or in need of comfort, you can learn to interpret their signals.

Some common newborn behaviors and their potential meanings are (*Newborn Behaviour*, 2022; Garoo, 2023; *Learning Your Baby's Cues*, n.d.):

- **Head banging:** This may be a self-soothing technique or a sign of frustration.
- **Constant kicking:** This could indicate gas, discomfort, or a desire to move and explore.
- **Turning the face away:** This may be a sign of overstimulation or a need for a break.
- **Arching back:** This may indicate discomfort, gas, or reflux.
- **Grumpiness:** This may be a sign of overtiredness, overstimulation, or hunger.
- **Fist clenching:** This could be a sign of hunger or stress.
- **Baby hiccups:** Common and usually harmless, may indicate a need to burp or be comforted.
- **Ear-grabbing:** This could be a sign of ear discomfort or an ear infection.
- **Eye-rubbing:** This could indicate tiredness or eye discomfort.
- **Grimacing, grunting, or bearing down:** This may indicate a need to pass stool or gas.
- **Breathing quickly:** This may be a sign of excitement, stress, or a need for a break.
- **Scrunching the knees:** This could indicate gas or digestive discomfort.
- **Sucking fingers:** This could be a sign of hunger or a self-soothing technique.
- **Arm jerks:** This may be a startle reflex or a sign of overstimulation.

Take some time to observe your baby and see if you can recognize any of these behaviors. The more you start to notice these cues, the quicker and easier it will be to respond to them.

Bonding With Your Baby

The bond between a baby and their caregiver is a strong emotional and physical connection that plays a vital role in the baby's overall well-being. This bonding process helps stimulate the production of hormones and chemicals in the brain that support the baby's brain growth and development (Pregnancy, Birth and Baby, n.d.). Bonding will also help create and strengthen connections between brain cells, laying the foundation for your baby's cognitive and emotional development.

It's important to note that while bonding is essential, it may not always happen instantly for every mother. Some moms may face challenges that can delay or hinder the bonding process, and it's important to note that this is more common than people realize, and it is *not* a reflection of your love for your baby.

Reasons why some moms may not bond with their baby right away include (Ayeni, 2023; Taylor, 2021):

- difficult delivery or postpartum complications
- struggling with breastfeeding challenges or feeling frustrated by difficulties
- dealing with postpartum depression or anxiety
- feeling exhausted and overwhelmed by the demands of new motherhood

- having a baby in the NICU, which can limit physical contact and interaction
- experiencing mood swings or hormonal changes that can impact emotional connection

Instant bonding is not always possible, and you shouldn't feel guilty about needing time to develop that connection if it doesn't happen right away. If you have concerns about bonding or are experiencing persistent feelings of detachment, discuss these concerns with a healthcare professional, such as your obstetrician, pediatrician, or a mental health provider specializing in perinatal care. They can offer support, guidance, and resources to help you navigate this challenging aspect of new motherhood.

Bonding With Your Baby During Feedings

Feeding time, whether through breastfeeding or bottle-feeding, provides a natural and intimate opportunity for bonding with your baby. It's important to remember that both methods of feeding can foster a strong connection between mother and child, and the decision to breastfeed or formula feed is a deeply personal one that should be respected and supported.

Breastfeeding promotes bonding through several means (*Breastfeeding and Bonding*, n.d.):

- **Skin-to-skin contact:** Holding your baby close during breastfeeding allows for direct skin-to-skin contact, which stimulates the release of oxytocin, also known as the "love hormone," in both mother and baby.

- **Comfort nursing:** Breastfeeding provides not only nourishment but also comfort and security for your baby, strengthening the emotional bond.
- **Scent and voice recognition:** During breastfeeding, your baby becomes familiar with your unique scent and voice, which can have a calming effect and reinforce the sense of attachment.
- **Increases sleepiness:** The hormones released during breastfeeding can help your baby feel sleepy and content, promoting a sense of relaxation and well-being.

It's worth noting that breastfeeding actually helps "promote mothering behaviors and the formation of a strong bond" due to the number of different hormones that are released (*Breastfeeding and Bonding,* n.d.).

Bottle-feeding can also be a valuable time for bonding, and there are several ways to promote connection during this experience (*How to Create a Special Bond When Bottle Feeding Your Baby*, 2023):

- **Hold your baby close:** Cuddle your baby while bottle-feeding, maintaining eye contact and physical closeness.
- **Talk and sing to your baby:** Engage with your baby through soft, soothing speech and gentle songs, which can help them feel secure and loved.

- **Practice skin-to-skin contact:** Remove your top and the baby's clothing to allow for direct skin-to-skin contact during bottle-feeding.
- **Take your time:** Bottle-feeding offers an opportunity to slow down and focus on your baby, enjoying the intimate bond you share.

Remember, regardless of your feeding choice, what matters most is the love, care, and attention you give to your baby during this special time. Trust your instincts, seek support when needed, and cherish the unique bond you are creating with your little one.

Talking to Your Baby

Talking to your baby is a simple yet powerful way to build a strong bond and support their language development. Even though your baby may not understand the words you say, they are constantly learning from your voice, facial expressions, and gestures.

Talking to your baby has numerous benefits. Exposure to language stimulates your baby's brain, helping to create neural connections that lay the foundation for future language skills (Kuhl, 2010). Engaging in conversation with your baby helps them feel loved, secure, and connected to you.

Babies learn to talk gradually, and their language development progresses through different stages:

- **1–3 months:** Cooing and gurgling.
- **4–7 months:** Babbling and imitating sounds.
- **8–12 months:** Saying first words and understanding simple phrases.

To make the most of your baby talk, keep these basics in mind:

- Make eye contact with your baby while speaking, as they respond better when looking directly at you.
- Talk with your baby as much as you can. It's true that talkative parents tend to have children who are the same.
- Engage in one-on-one conversations with your baby without distractions from other adults or children.
- When your baby tries to talk back to you, show interest and encourage them by listening attentively.
- Incorporate adult speech patterns alongside baby talk to help your baby learn how words sound in everyday conversation.
- Limit your baby's exposure to TV, as too much can hinder language growth.

Here are some fun and effective ways to talk to your baby (Taylor, n.d.-a; Weiss, 2021):

- Label objects, people, and emotions to help your baby associate words with their meanings.
- Ask questions and pause for your baby's response, even if they can't answer yet.

- Play with pitch and intonation to capture your baby's attention.
- Narrate your day, describing your actions and surroundings.
- Read books together, pointing at pictures and discussing the story.
- Embrace animal sounds and other playful vocalizations.
- Mimic your baby's babbling to encourage back-and-forth conversation.
- Sing songs and rhymes to make language learning enjoyable.
- Listen attentively as your baby practices new sounds and words.
- Most importantly, have fun and enjoy the process of communicating with your little one!
- Know when to take a break if your baby becomes overstimulated or disinterested.

Baby Massage

A Baby massage is a wonderful way to bond with your little one while providing numerous physical and emotional benefits. The gentle, nurturing touch of a massage can help promote relaxation, improve sleep, and enhance communication between parent and child. Other benefits include (Children's Hospital of Richmond at VCU, 2017):

- strengthening the parent-child bond through physical touch and focused attention

- promoting relaxation and reducing stress for both baby and parent
- improving sleep quality and duration
- supporting healthy growth and development
- easing common discomforts such as colic, gas, and constipation

Here are some simple massage techniques to try with your baby:

- **Water wheel:** Place your hands on your baby's chest and gently move them down the body, one after the other, as if forming a water wheel.
- **Milking the leg:** Gently squeeze and release your baby's legs, working from the thigh to the ankle.
- **Open book:** With your baby on their back, gently "open" their chest by moving their arms outward and then inward, as if opening a book.
- **"I love you":** On your baby's tummy, trace the words "I," "L," and "U" using gentle strokes.
- **Sun and moon:** Make circular motions on your baby's tummy with your hands, one clockwise (sun) and the other counterclockwise (moon).

When giving your baby a massage, keep these safety tips in mind:

- Use a safe, edible oil suitable for your baby's delicate skin, such as coconut, almond, or jojoba oil.
- Always support your baby's wrist or ankle with one hand while massaging their arms or legs.

- When making circular motions on your baby's tummy, go clockwise to follow the natural direction of digestion.
- Stop massaging if your baby becomes upset or falls asleep, respecting their cues and comfort level.

Incorporating a massage into your daily routine can help you foster a deeper connection and promote your baby's overall well-being.

Bonding With Your Baby During Bath Time

Bath time is not only essential for keeping your baby clean and healthy but also provides a wonderful opportunity for bonding and creating special memories together. This intimate, one-on-one time allows you to focus solely on your baby without distractions, fostering a deeper connection.

Bath time is a tech-free zone, allowing you to be fully present with your little one without the interruptions of phones, TV, or other devices. It also helps establish a consistent routine, which can be comforting and reassuring for babies.

Here are some ways you can use bath time to bond with your baby:

- **Actively play together:** Use bath toys, gentle splashing, and playful interactions to engage your baby and make bath time fun.
- **Have heart-to-heart conversations:** Talk softly to your baby, maintaining eye contact and expressing your love and affection.

- **Sing lullabies together:** Soothe your baby with gentle songs and melodies, creating a calming and nurturing atmosphere.
- **Keep safety in mind:** Always prioritize your baby's safety by ensuring the water temperature is appropriate, supporting their head and neck, and never leaving them unattended.
- **Read bath books together:** Introduce waterproof books to stimulate your baby's senses and promote early literacy skills.
- **Tap into physical touch:** Use gentle strokes, massages, and cuddles to provide comfort and strengthen your bond through physical connection.
- **Chat and learn:** Describe your actions and name body parts as you bathe your baby, promoting language development and body awareness.

To properly bathe your newborn, follow these steps:

1. Gather all necessary supplies before starting.
2. Fill the tub or sink with 2–3 inches of warm water (around 100 °F/38 °C).
3. Gently lower your baby into the water, supporting their head and neck.
4. Use a soft washcloth or sponge to clean your baby, starting with the face and working your way down.
5. Pay special attention to creases and folds in the skin, as these areas can easily harbor bacteria.
6. Gently wash your baby's hair with a mild, tear-free shampoo.

7. Rinse your baby thoroughly, remove them from the water, and immediately wrap them in a soft, warm towel.

Focusing on bonding and safety during bath time will help you create a special ritual that promotes closeness and creates lasting memories for both you and your little one.

Bonding With Your Baby During Play Time

Play time is a crucial aspect of your baby's development and provides an excellent opportunity for bonding and strengthening your connection. Engaging in age-appropriate play activities with your baby not only supports their cognitive, physical, and emotional growth but also fosters a deep sense of love and trust between you and your little one.

Through play, babies learn about the world around them, develop new skills, and build confidence. When you actively participate in your baby's play time, you create a safe and nurturing environment that encourages exploration, learning, and the development of a strong, loving relationship. Let's look at some age-appropriate ways to play with your baby (*Playtime With Your Baby*, 2022; Stewart, 2023; *Thinking and Play: Babies*, 2022):

3–6 months

- Engage in face-to-face interactions, making eye contact and smiling.
- Play peek-a-boo to encourage object permanence and social skills.

- Provide soft, textured toys for sensory exploration.
- Sing songs and nursery rhymes to promote language development.

6–9 months

- Introduce simple cause-and-effect toys, such as stackable rings or balls.
- Play gentle chase or crawling games to encourage physical development.
- Engage in simple pretend play, like talking on a toy phone.
- Read colorful board books together, pointing out pictures and naming objects.

9–12 months

- Offer problem-solving toys, such as shape sorters or simple puzzles.
- Play hide-and-seek or other games that involve taking turns.
- Encourage imitation and pretend play with dolls, toy cars, or play kitchens.
- Dance and sing to music together, fostering rhythm and coordination.

The most important aspect of playtime is your presence and engagement. When you give your undivided attention, show enthusiasm, and follow your baby's lead, you create a strong foundation for bonding and learning.

Baby Milestone

Documenting your baby's milestones is a wonderful way to preserve precious memories and celebrate the incredible growth and development that occurs during the first year of life. Not only does it provide a tangible record of your child's progress, but it also allows you to reflect on your own journey as a parent and the love and care you've poured into nurturing your little one.

There are many reasons to document your baby's milestones:

- It creates a cherished keepsake that you and your child can look back on for years to come.
- It helps you recognize and celebrate the significant moments and achievements in your baby's life.
- It provides an opportunity for you to reflect on your own growth and progress as a parent.
- It allows you to share your child's development with family and friends who may not be able to witness these moments in person.

There are several options for creating a baby milestone keepsake, depending on your preferences and creativity:

- **Baby milestone board:** Create a DIY milestone board using a lightweight board, printable milestone cards or stickers, and decorative elements. Arrange the cards on the board and update it with photos as your baby reaches each milestone.

- **Baby's first-year memory book:** Purchase a pre-made memory book or create your own using a scrapbook or photo album. Fill the pages with photos, milestone stickers, and written reflections on your baby's development and your own experiences as a parent.
- **Milestone blanket or cards:** Use a milestone blanket or cards that feature pre-printed milestone markers, such as monthly age or significant achievements. Take photos of your baby with the corresponding milestone marker and create a photo series or collage.
- **Digital milestone tracking:** Use a digital app or platform to track and document your baby's milestones. Many apps allow you to add photos, videos, and written reflections, and some even provide personalized development insights and tips.

Whichever method you choose, the key is to be consistent and make it a fun, enjoyable process. Set aside time each month or after significant milestones to update your keepsake and reflect on the incredible journey you and your baby are on together.

Remember, documenting your baby's milestones isn't just about creating a beautiful keepsake; it's also an opportunity to celebrate the wonder and joy of your child's growth and development. As you look back on these moments in the years to come, you'll be reminded of the incredible love and strength that defines your journey as a parent.

Journal Prompts

As you know, journaling can help you capture and reflect on your precious experiences with your baby. Allow yourself some space to ponder how you will strengthen your bond with your baby:

- What has been the most surprising aspect of bonding with your baby? How has your relationship evolved since their birth?
- Describe a moment of pure joy you experienced with your baby this week. What made that moment so special, and how did it make you feel as a mother?
- Reflect on a challenging moment you faced with your baby recently. How did you handle it, and what did you learn about yourself and your baby through that experience?
- Write a letter to your baby, expressing your hopes, dreams, and promises for your future together. What kind of mother do you aspire to be, and what values do you hope to instill in your child?
- Imagine yourself one year from now, looking back on this time with your newborn. What advice would you give to your current self? What do you want to remember about this special time in your life?

Key Takeaways and What's Next

Here, we explored the essential elements of newborn bonding and how to nurture the special connection between mother and baby. We learned that creating a strong, loving bond with your baby is crucial for their emotional and mental development. When we engage in bonding activities like skin-to-skin contact, breastfeeding or bottle-feeding, talking and singing to your baby, and participating in age-appropriate play, we lay the foundation for a secure attachment and healthy development.

As you continue on your motherhood journey, I want you to prioritize creating moments of connection with your baby through daily routines like feeding, bathing, and playtime. Embrace the power of touch, eye contact, and verbal communication to strengthen your bond. Remember, you are your baby's first and most important teacher, and the love and attention you provide during these early months will have a lasting impact on their development and your relationship.

Looking ahead, Chapter 10 will focus on the importance of nourishing connections with others during the postpartum period. While the bond with your baby is undeniably special, it's also essential to cultivate supportive relationships with your partner, family, friends, and fellow mothers.

Part V: Thriving as a Woman and a Mom

Building Your Village—Nurturing Connections in Motherhood

Don't underestimate the importance of having a support system—it can truly be a game-changer for your well-being and confidence as a new parent.

Allison Banfield

While motherhood truly is a beautiful journey, it can also feel overwhelming, challenging, and, at times, isolating. Having a strong, supportive community can help you feel more connected, empowered, and capable.

In this chapter, we'll discuss the value of building a supportive village and the various ways you can nurture connections with others during your postpartum journey. While the bond between mother and child is undeniably special, it's equally important to work on your relationships with your partner, family, friends, and even fellow mothers. These connections can provide you with the emotional support, practical help, and sense of belonging that are essential for thriving in motherhood.

Connecting With Your Partner

Having a baby can significantly impact a couple's relationship, bringing both joy and new challenges. Common issues that arise in a partnership after welcoming a child include doubled domestic duties, conflicting parenting styles, decreased intimacy and sex, limited couple time, lack of personal time, and financial concerns.

Adjusting to parenthood takes time, patience, and effort from both partners. In order to strengthen your bond with your partner after giving birth, consider using the following strategies:

- **Discuss parenting views:** Openly communicate about your parenting philosophy, values, and expectations to ensure you're on the same page.
- **Spend time as a couple:** Prioritize regular date nights or quality time together, even if it's just a few minutes each day.
- **Don't forget self-care:** Encourage each other to engage in individual self-care activities to maintain personal well-being and reduce stress.
- **Discuss finances:** Have honest conversations about money, budgeting, and financial goals to avoid misunderstandings and work together as a team.

- **Ask for support:** Be open about your needs and ask for help from your partner, whether it's with household chores, childcare, or emotional support.
- **Check-in daily:** Make a habit of checking in with each other daily, sharing your thoughts, feelings, and experiences.
- **Talk about your dreams:** Discuss your individual and shared dreams for the future, ensuring that you continue to grow together as a couple.
- **Have sex:** When you feel ready, prioritize physical intimacy and explore new ways to connect sexually that work for your current situation.
- **Communicate:** Practice open, honest, and respectful communication, actively listening to each other and expressing your needs and feelings clearly.

Connecting With Friends

Becoming a parent can significantly impact friendships as priorities shift and time becomes more limited. Some friends may not understand the demands of motherhood, leading to potential conflicts or distance in relationships. To help you navigate these changes, you can try the following tips:

- Nurture existing relationships by staying in touch, even if it's just a quick text or phone call.
- Accept that quality time with friends may look different now, such as shorter visits or including your baby.
- Utilize video calls to stay connected when in-person meetups are challenging.

- Connect with other moms who can provide support, advice, and companionship.
- Be open to making new friends who are in a similar life stage and can relate to your experiences.
- Invite friends over to your home, where you can socialize in a comfortable environment while tending to your baby's needs.
- Make an effort to attend your friends' important events and celebrations, even if you can only stay for a short while.

True friends will understand and support you through this transitional period. Be honest about your needs and limitations and cherish the friendships that adapt and grow with you.

Building Your Support Network

Having a strong support network is crucial for new mothers during the postpartum period. New motherhood can be a demanding and overwhelming time, and having support can make a significant difference in a mother's well-being. Postpartum support can come in various forms, such as emotional support, practical help with daily tasks, or even just having someone to talk to. Your postpartum support network can also serve as an extra set of eyes and ears, helping you identify any potential issues or concerns.

The first step in building your support network is to identify the tasks you'll need help with after your baby is born, such as *(3 Steps to Building Your Postpartum Support Network, n.d.)*:

- **Physical support:** This includes tasks such as cooking, cleaning, caring for your child or children, grocery shopping or other errands, and taking you for a walk or to an appointment.
- **Emotional support:** This includes sitting with and listening to you, offering affection, giving encouraging words, praying, or even meditating with you.

Name the people who can help with these tasks. Consider both physical and emotional supporters, and don't hesitate to think outside your inner circle.

Once you've done that, you can match people with specific postpartum jobs based on their abilities, availability, and your level of comfort with them. This is an ongoing process, so be open to first accepting help, and also communicating your needs clearly. Surround yourself with people who uplift and encourage you during this time. Whether it's family, friends, or professionals, having a strong support system can help you navigate the challenges of motherhood with greater ease and confidence.

Spiritual Connection

For many new mothers, the journey into motherhood is not just a physical and emotional experience but also a deeply spiritual one. The act of bringing new life into the world can evoke a profound sense of connection to something greater than oneself. Embracing the spiritual significance of motherhood can provide a sense of purpose, meaning, and resilience during the postpartum period.

Spirituality can offer numerous benefits for postpartum health, such as reducing stress, promoting emotional well-being, and fostering a sense of inner peace (Backes et al., 2022). Engaging in spiritual practices can help new mothers navigate the challenges of this time with greater clarity, compassion, and strength.

Here are some tips for nurturing your spiritual connection during the postpartum period:

- **Sound bath:** Participate in a sound bath or listen to soothing music that resonates with your spirit. The vibrations and harmonies can promote deep relaxation and emotional balance.
- **Nature therapy:** Spend time in nature, whether it's taking a walk in the park, sitting by a lake, or gardening. Connecting with the natural world can be grounding and restorative.
- **Movement medicine:** Engage in mindful movement practices like yoga, tai chi, or dance. These activities can help you connect with your body, release tension, and find a sense of flow and harmony.

Spiritual Meditation

A spiritual meditation practice can help you connect with your higher self and find inner peace during the postpartum period. Here's a simple guided meditation to try:

1. Find a quiet, comfortable space. Look for somewhere you can sit or lie down without being distracted.
2. Close your eyes and take a few deep breaths. Your body should relax into stillness.
3. Bring your awareness to your breath, noticing the sensation of the air moving in and out of your lungs.
4. As you inhale, imagine drawing in positive energy, love, and light. As you exhale, release any tension, worries, or negative thoughts.
5. Continue this breathing pattern, allowing yourself to sink deeper into a state of relaxation and inner connection.
6. When you feel ready, gently open your eyes and take a moment to appreciate the sense of peace and clarity you've cultivated.

Journal Prompts

How will you nurture connections in your life? Consider the following:

- What does spirituality mean to you, and how has your spiritual perspective shifted since becoming a mother?
- Reflect on a moment of deep connection or transcendence you've experienced recently. What insights or lessons did you gain from this experience?
- Write a letter of gratitude to the universe, acknowledging the blessings and challenges of your motherhood journey.

- Imagine your highest, most compassionate self. What advice or wisdom would she offer you in this moment?
- Set an intention for your spiritual growth as a mother. What practices or habits do you want to cultivate to support your inner journey?

Key Takeaways and What's Next

In this chapter, we have considered the importance of building a supportive village and nurturing connections during the postpartum period. We discussed the various ways to strengthen your relationship with your partner, navigate changes in friendships, and create a postpartum support network that meets your physical and emotional needs.

We have discovered that taking care of yourself and investing in your relationships is crucial for thriving in motherhood. Remember, asking for help is a sign of strength, not weakness. It's okay to reach out for support and seek resources that can help you navigate the challenges of the postpartum period. Whether it's joining a mothers group, hiring a postpartum doula or lactation consultant, or seeking guidance from a therapist, there are numerous ways to expand your network of support.

As you continue on your motherhood journey, prioritize self-care and make time for practices that nourish your mind, body, and spirit. Engage in activities that bring you joy, promote relaxation, and help you feel more connected to yourself and others.

Our final chapter will focus on finding balance and harmony between motherhood and other aspects of your life.

ELEVEN

Harmonizing Life–Balancing Motherhood With Personal Growth

A strong mom knows the power of self-care and seeks to nourish her own well-being, enabling her to better care for others.

Elizabeth Gilbert

B eing a mother is one of the most rewarding and fulfilling roles, but it is also one of the most demanding. Juggling the responsibilities of caring for a child while also pursuing personal growth and maintaining a sense of self can feel like an overwhelming task. However, through the power of self-care and the deliberate nourishment of one's own well-being, a mother can find the strength and resilience needed to balance these many facets of life.

In this chapter, we will explore the strategies and insights needed to harmonize the beautiful chaos of motherhood with the essential pursuit of personal growth. One of the most common challenges we face as new mothers is the feeling of losing ourselves in the all-consuming role of parenthood. It can be easy to get swept up in the constant demands of caring for a child and neglect our own needs and desires. We might even believe that taking care of ourselves is selfish, but I want you to remember that it is a necessary component of being a strong and capable mother.

Finding Your Passion and Hobbies

As a mom, it's easy to get caught up in the daily responsibilities of caring for your children and managing your household. However, pursuing your own passions and hobbies is crucial for maintaining a sense of self and finding fulfillment outside of your role as a mother.

Engaging in hobbies has many benefits for you as a mom. Firstly, they **enhance socialization** by providing opportunities to connect with others who share similar interests, helping you build a supportive network outside of your family. Pursuing hobbies also **nurtures your individual interests**, allowing you to maintain a sense of individuality and explore interests that are separate from your identity as a mother. Engaging in enjoyable activities can also help **alleviate the stress and pressure** that often accompany parenting responsibilities.

Moreover, cultivating hobbies now can help you **build a fulfilling life outside of motherhood**, making the transition easier when your children eventually leave home. By prioritizing your own interests and self-care, you **teach your children** the importance of maintaining mental well-being and pursuing personal growth. Additionally, hobbies present **opportunities for continuous learning**, enabling you to learn new skills, engage your mind, and satisfy your natural curiosity.

If you're not sure where to start, consider exploring some of these fun hobby ideas:

- reading or joining a book club
- practicing yoga or meditation
- crafting DIY projects
- gardening
- cooking or baking
- engaging in fitness activities or dancing
- taking online courses
- writing or journaling
- starting a blog
- painting or drawing
- learning pottery

The key is to find activities that bring you joy and provide a sense of accomplishment. Don't be afraid to try new things and experiment until you discover hobbies that resonate with you.

Managing Work and Motherhood

Balancing the demands of motherhood and a career can be very challenging, but with the right strategies and support, it is possible to find harmony between these two important roles. Here are some tips to help you navigate the balancing act of being a working mom (Miller, n.d.):

- **Choose a family-friendly employer:** Seek out companies that offer policies and benefits that support working parents, such as flexible schedules, remote work options, or childcare assistance.
- **Set a routine:** Establish a consistent schedule for your work and family responsibilities to create structure and predictability in your daily life.
- **Work efficiently:** Streamline your work processes, delegate when possible, and eliminate unnecessary distractions to maximize your productivity during work hours.
- **Prioritize tasks:** Focus on the most important and time-sensitive tasks first, both at work and at home, to ensure that you're making the most of your time and energy.
- **Make the most of your commute:** Use your travel time to catch up on emails, plan your day, or engage in self-care activities like listening to podcasts or practicing mindfulness.
- **Set and keep boundaries:** Communicate your needs and limitations clearly to your employer and family and be consistent in upholding the boundaries you set to protect your well-being and work-life balance.
- **Be fully present:** When you're at work, give your full attention to your job, and when you're with your family, put away work-related thoughts and focus on enjoying quality time with your loved ones.

- **Outsource chores:** Consider hiring help for household tasks or delegating chores to family members to free up more time for work and family commitments.
- **Reevaluate other commitments:** Assess your involvement in activities outside of work and family and consider scaling back on those that don't align with your priorities or bring you joy.
- **Get enough sleep:** Prioritize rest to ensure that you have the energy and focus needed to manage your work and family responsibilities effectively.
- **Enjoy time for yourself:** Carve out moments for self-care and pursuing your own interests, as this will help you recharge and be a better mother and employee.
- **Soak in the snuggles:** Cherish the special moments with your children, as they serve as a reminder of the importance of your role as a mother and the joy it brings to your life.

Finding the right balance between motherhood and career is an ongoing process that requires flexibility, adaptability, and self-compassion. These strategies will help you navigate the challenges of being a working mom, and help you find fulfillment in both your professional and personal life.

Rediscovering Yourself

It's common for new mothers to feel like they've lost a sense of their identity after having a baby. The all-consuming nature of motherhood can make it challenging to prioritize one's own needs and interests. However, rediscovering yourself after motherhood is crucial not only for your own well-being but also for setting a positive example for your children. Your dreams, aspirations, and goals still matter, and finding a balance between your role as a mother and your individual identity is essential.

One way to do this is by stepping back from the constant stream of social media and turning inward to your own thoughts, emotions, and experiences. By challenging negative self-talk and reframing your mindset, you can open up new possibilities for self-discovery. Reflecting on your core values, interests, and personal goals can provide clarity on what truly matters to you.

A powerful question to think about is this: "If you woke up tomorrow, and your life was exactly how you wanted it to be, what would that ideal life look like?" This exercise can help you realize your deepest desires and aspirations, guiding you toward setting achievable short-term and long-term goals for yourself. Prioritizing self-care activities that cater to your mental, physical, and spiritual well-being is essential in nurturing your overall self.

Taking a leisurely stroll outdoors can help clear your mind and foster a connection with nature, providing a calming break from your daily responsibilities. Even the simple act of getting dressed each day, transitioning from pajamas to your favorite clothes, can uplift your spirits and boost your confidence. It can also really help to revisit activities and hobbies that brought you joy before motherhood.

Also, don't hesitate to step out of the house for some personal time, whether it's attending a class or catching up with a friend over coffee. Finally, embrace this new chapter of your life without comparing it to your pre-motherhood self; instead, see it as an opportunity for growth, self-discovery, and embracing the evolving layers of your identity.

Rediscovering yourself after motherhood is a journey, and it may take time and effort to find the right balance. Be patient with yourself and celebrate the small victories along the way as you navigate this new chapter in your life. Here are some tips to help you balance being a mom and being yourself:

- Accept that motherhood is now a part of your identity, but it doesn't define your entire being.
- Make time for adult conversations and interactions to stimulate your mind and maintain a sense of self.
- Indulge in a passion or hobby that brings you joy and fulfillment.
- Let go of the guilt associated with taking time for yourself.
- Transform nap times into "me time" to pursue your own interests or practice self-care.
- Don't neglect your own needs; a happy and fulfilled mother is better equipped to care for her family.

Journal Prompts

Finding balance in motherhood is a constant challenge. Sometimes we need to be reminded to prioritize our own well-being. How about taking some time this week to reflect on how you want to achieve this balance? The following prompts are designed to help you set some goals and intentions:

- What activities or moments in your life bring you the most joy and fulfillment?
- Describe a time when you felt truly proud of yourself. What qualities or strengths did you exhibit in that moment?
- If you could spend an entire day doing anything you wanted without any constraints, what would you choose to do?
- Write about a challenge you've faced as a mother and how overcoming it has helped you grow and discover new aspects of yourself.
- What are three things you're deeply passionate about, and how can you incorporate them into your life in a meaningful way?
- Imagine yourself in five years. What does your ideal life look like, and what steps can you take now to start moving toward that vision?
- Reflect on a moment of self-discovery you experienced recently. What did you learn about yourself, and how has that knowledge impacted your perspective?
- Write a love letter to yourself, celebrating your unique qualities, strengths, and accomplishments.
- What limiting beliefs or fears hold you back from pursuing your passions? How can you reframe these thoughts in a more empowering light?

- Describe your ideal day as a mother and as an individual. How can you create more moments that align with this vision in your daily life?

Key Takeaways and What's Next

Throughout this chapter, we've explored the importance of balancing motherhood with personal growth and self-discovery. We've discussed the value of pursuing passions and hobbies, managing the demands of work and family life, and rediscovering yourself amidst the transformative journey of motherhood.

We have learned that prioritizing self-care and personal growth is not selfish; it's essential for being the best mother and woman you can be. So carve out time for your own interests, set boundaries, and accept your unique identity.

Finding this balance between being a strong mother and an unstoppable woman is incredibly empowering. It allows you to model self-love, resilience, and the pursuit of dreams for your children while also nurturing your own well-being and sense of purpose. Remember, a happy and fulfilled mother is better equipped to handle the challenges of motherhood and create a thriving, loving home environment.

As we come to the end of this book, let's take a moment to reflect on everything we've discussed together. From understanding the profound changes of motherhood to prioritizing self-care, building a support network, and finding harmony between your roles, each chapter has provided insights and strategies to help you navigate this wonderful time of your life with grace, resilience, and joy.

Thank you for choosing this book as your companion on your motherhood journey. By investing in yourself and your well-being, you're not only creating a better life for yourself but also laying the foundation for a more fulfilling and connected experience with your child. Remember, you are exactly the mother your child needs, and your love, strength, and dedication are shaping their world in countless beautiful ways.

As you move forward, carry these lessons and insights with you, and continue to prioritize your own growth and happiness. Surround yourself with supportive people, practice self-compassion, and embrace the magic and messiness of motherhood. Most importantly, trust in your own inner wisdom and know that you have everything you need to thrive as a mother and as a woman.

The journey of motherhood is an ongoing one, filled with joys, challenges, and opportunities for growth. May you continue to find strength, purpose, and fulfillment in this incredible role, and may the lessons and strategies shared in this book serve as a guiding light as you navigate the beautiful, complex, and rewarding path of being a mother.

Conclusion

We have a secret in our culture, and it's not that birth is painful. It's that women are strong.

Laura Stavoe Harm

Wow, what an incredible journey we've taken together! We've discussed the joys of the postpartum period as well as the challenges, and we've highlighted the absolute strength that lies within every mother.

The path of motherhood is not easy, but it is a path that reveals the incredible resilience and power that resides within each and every one of us. Whether you're navigating the early days of postpartum recovery, finding your footing as a new mother, or rediscovering yourself during the beautiful chaos of parenthood, please know that you are not alone. The experiences, insights, and strategies we have shared here are a sign of the collective wisdom and strength of mothers everywhere.

If there is one message that you take away from this book, let it be this one:

You are exactly the mother your child needs, and you have everything that you need to thrive on this journey within you.

When you can prioritize self-care, build a supportive network, and embrace the unique strengths and challenges of your motherhood experience, you can cultivate a sense of confidence, resilience, and joy that will carry you through even the toughest of times.

As you close this book, take a moment to acknowledge what an incredible feat you have accomplished: You have grown, nurtured, and brought forth a new life into this world. You have faced the depths of exhaustion, the heights of love, and everything in between. You are a warrior, a nurturer, and a force to be reckoned with.

So, as you move forward on this journey of motherhood, remember to believe in yourself and the incredible strength that lies within you. Use all of the tools and strategies you've learned that work for you and know that you have the power to create a beautiful, fulfilling life for yourself and your family. You already are a brave and unstoppable woman, and with these tools, you'll be able to face anything that comes your way.

Take care of yourself, dear mama.

Make a Difference ~ Please Leave a Review

My mission is to bring the importance of postpartum self-care to every family. But I can only fulfill that mission by reaching parents like you.

This is where you can help! People often judge a book by its cover—and its reviews. So, if you've found value in the words and wisdom shared within these pages, please consider leaving a review.

Your feedback helps other moms find the support and guidance they need on this incredible journey. Your words could help...

- One more mom feel less overwhelmed and isolated
- One more parent find peace during the postpartum period
- One more family gain the strength to thrive during those tough early days
- One more woman to be empowered and gain confidence in her journey
- One more dream of a balanced and fulfilling motherhood become a reality

Simply scan the QR code below to share your thoughts:

Thank you from the bottom of my heart.

Warmly,
Ava Wells

References

Alpert, Y. M. (2022, January 3). *What to expect emotionally after birth.* The Bump. https://www.thebump.com/a/postpartum-feelings-to-expect#2

Anokye, R., Acheampong, E., Budu-Ainooson, A., Obeng, E. I., & Akwasi, A. G. (2018). Prevalence of postpartum depression and interventions utilized for its management. *Annals of General Psychiatry, 17*(1). https://doi.org/10.1186/s12991-018-0188-0

Ayeni, A. (2023, December 13). *Mother-Infant bonding: It's not always instant.* Postpartum Support International (PSI). https://www.postpartum.net/mother-infant-bonding-its-not-always-instant/

Backes, D. S., Gomes, E. B., Rangel, R. F., Rolim, K. M. C., Arrusul, L. S., & Abaid, J. L. W. (2022). Meaning of the spiritual aspects of health care in pregnancy and childbirth. *Rev Lat Am Enfermagem., 30.* https://doi.org/10.1590/1518-8345.5980.3774

Better Health Channel. (n.d.). *Breastfeeding—mastitis and other nipple and breast problems.* https://www.betterhealth.vic.gov.au/health/healthyliving/breastfeeding-mastitis-and-other-nipple-and-breast-problems

Breastcancer.org. (2024, April 5). *Breast self-exam.* https://www.breastcancer.org/screening-testing/breast-self-exam-bse

Breast Cancer Now. (n.d.). *Breast changes during or after pregnancy.* https://breastcancernow.org/about-breast-cancer/breast-lumps-and-benign-not-cancer-breast-conditions/breast-changes-during-or-after-pregnancy/

Breastfeeding and bonding. (n.d.). Byram Healthcare. https://breastpumps.byramhealthcare.com/blog/2018/11/23/breastfeeding-bonding

Britt, T. (2022, March 29). *What vaginal changes can a person expect after giving birth?* MedicalNewsToday. https://www.medicalnewstoday.com/articles/vagina-after-giving-birth#urinary-incontinence

Brown, T. (n.d.). *8 mindset strategies to psychologically prepare for birth.* Dr Tess Browne. https://drtessbrowne.com/journal/8-mindset-strategies-to-psychologically-prepare-for-birth

Can a mother be iron-deficient while breastfeeding? (n.d.). Vinmec. https://www.vinmec.com/en/news/health-news/obstetrics-gynecology-and-assisted-reproductive-technologies-art/can-a-mother-be-iron-deficient-while-breastfeeding/

Care of your breasts. (n.d.). The Society of Obstetricians and Gynaecologists of Canada. https://www.pregnancyinfo.ca/postpartum/postpartum/care-of-your-breasts/

Centers for Disease Control and Prevention [CDC]. (2024, February 26). *Alcohol.* https://www.cdc.gov/breastfeeding/breastfeeding-special-circum stances/vaccinations-medications-drugs/alcohol.html#:~

CDC. (2024, February 19). *Maternal diet and breastfeeding.* https://www.cdc. gov/breastfeeding/breastfeeding-special-circumstances/diet-and-micronu trients/maternal-diet.html#:~

Chen, Y., Michalak, M., & Agellon, L. B. (2018). Importance of nutrients and nutrient metabolism on human health. *The Yale Journal of Biology and Medicine, 91*(2), 95–103. https://www.ncbi.nlm.nih.gov/pmc/articles/ PMC6020734/

Children's Hospital of Richmond at VCU. (2017, February 1). *The many benefits of infant massage.* https://www.chrichmond.org/blog/the-many-bene fits-of-infant-massage#:~

Cleveland Clinic. (n.d.). *Aerobic exercise.* https://my.clevelandclinic.org/ health/articles/7050-aerobic-exercise

Cleveland Clinic. (2018). *Pregnancy: Physical changes after delivery.* https:// my.clevelandclinic.org/health/articles/9682-pregnancy-physical-changes-after-delivery

Colino, S., & Fabian-Weber, N. (2023, August 24). *We need to talk about postpartum anxiety.* Parents. https://www.parents.com/parenting/moms/ healthy-mom/the-other-postpartum-problem-anxiety/

Cruz, P. *Penelope Cruz quotes.* BrainyQuote. https://www.brainyquote.com/ quotes/penelope_cruz_542224

Depression in pregnant women and mothers: How children are affected. (2004). *Paediatrics & Child Health, 9*(8), 584–586. https://doi.org/10.1093/ pch/9.8.584

Dewar, G. (2022, June). *Postpartum stress: A guide for the science-minded parent.* Parenting Science. https://parentingscience.com/postpartum-stress/

Diet for breastfeeding mothers. (n.d.). The Children's Hospital of Philadelphia. https://www.chop.edu/pages/diet-breastfeeding-mothers#:~

Dipple, J. (n.d.). *Postpartum depression quotes.* Goodreads. https://www. goodreads.com/quotes/tag/postpartum-depression

Familydoctor.org editorial staff. (2017, April 7). *Postpartum depression* (PPD). Familydoctor.org. https://familydoctor.org/condition/postpartum-depres sion/

Firth, J., Gangwisch, J. E., Borisini, A., Wootton, R. E., & Mayer, E. A. (2020). Food and mood: How do diet and nutrition affect mental wellbeing? *BMJ*, *369*(1). https://doi.org/10.1136/bmj.m2382

Fowler, P. (n.d.). *Breathing techniques for stress relief.* WebMD. https://www.webmd.com/balance/stress-management/stress-relief-breathing-tech niques

Fox, I. (2023, June 24). *5 exercises to try after a C-section.* Parents. https://www.parents.com/pregnancy/giving-birth/cesarean/post-c-section-strengthening-exercises/

Freutel, N. (2018, October 5). *5 exercises to help with your C-section recovery.* Healthline. https://www.healthline.com/health/pregnancy/C-section-recovery-exercises

Garoo, R. (2023, November 3). *14 different baby cues and what they mean.* MomJunction. https://www.momjunction.com/articles/newborn-baby-body-language-cues-meaning_00698263/

Geisinger. (n.d.). *Postpartum care for mom: Tips for healing and comfort.* https://www.geisinger.org/patient-care/conditions-treatments-specialty/self-care-during-the-postpartum-period

Gilbert, E. (n.d.). Quote in Almer, C. (2023, August 1). *Empowering and inspiring: Top 20 strong mom quotes for unstoppable women.* Blinkest Magazine. www.blinkist.com/magazine/posts/empowering-inspiring-top-20-strong-mom-quotes-unstoppable-women?utm_source=cpp

Global Self-Care Federation. (n.d.). *What is self-care?* https://www.selfcarefed eration.org/what-is-self-care

Hagen, B. (2018, December 7). *10 ways your body changes after pregnancy.* Baptist Health. https://www.baptist-health.com/blog/10-ways-your-body-changes-after-pregnancy/

Harm, L. S. (n.d.). Quote in Dr. Laura (2019, August 26). *60 inspirational quotes for new moms.* St Johns Pediatric Dentistry. https://stjohnskids.com/blog/inspirational-quotes-about-becoming-a-mother-for-the-first-time/

HealthLink BC. (2013, August 5). *Vaginal care after giving birth.* https://www.healthlinkbc.ca/pregnancy-parenting/labour-and-birth/after-labour-and-care-new-moms/vaginal-care-after-giving-birth

Horsager-Boehrer, R. (2022, October 11). *6 ways to embrace a more positive body image during and after pregnancy.* UT Southwestern Medical Center. https://utswmed.org/medblog/perinatal-body-dissatisfaction/#:~

Hoshaw, C. (2022, March 29). *What is mindfulness? A simple practice for greater well-being*. Healthline. https://www.healthline.com/health/mind-body/what-is-mindfulness

How to create a special bond when bottle feeding your baby. (2023, November 27). PBC BABY Expo. https://pbcexpo.com.au/news/how-to-create-a-special-bond-when-bottle-feeding-your-baby

Huff, C. (n.d.). Quote in Tingley, L. (2021, August 29). *45 tired mom quotes every exhausted mom needs to hear*. Simply Well Balanced. https://simply-well-balanced.com/tired-mom-quotes/

Hughes, M. (n.d.). *Tips for proper hydration during pregnancy and postpartum workouts*. Dr Mae Hughes. https://drmaehughes.com/2023/04/28/hydrate-to-elevate-how-proper-hydration-enhances-pregnancy-and-postpartum-workouts/

Johnson, K. (n.d.). Quote in Kate. (n.d.). *23 powerful postpartum body quotes*. Mom With Anxiety. https://momwithanxiety.com/postpartum-body-quotes/

Joy, A. (n.d.). Quote in Bradley, J. (2020, June 3). *25 postpartum fitness quotes to motivate new moms*. Dr. Jena Bradley. https://livecorestrong.com/postpartum-fitness-quotes/

Juber, B. A., Jackson, K. H., Johnson, K. B., Harris, W. S., & Baack, M. L. (2016). Breast milk DHA levels may increase after informing women: A community-based cohort study from South Dakota USA. *International Breastfeeding Journal, 12*(1). https://doi.org/10.1186/s13006-016-0099-0

Kate. (n.d.). *23 powerful postpartum body quotes*. Mom With Anxiety. https://momwithanxiety.com/postpartum-body-quotes/

Keeping hydrated during pregnancy and the postpartum period. (2022, July 18). Stork Helpers. https://www.storkhelpers.com/blog/entry/keeping-hydrated-during-pregnancy-and-the-postpartum-period/#:~

Kingsolver, B. (n.d.). *Barbara Kingslover quotes*. Goodreads. https://www.goodreads.com/quotes/27874-sometimes-the-strength-of-motherhood-is-greater-than-natural-laws

Kripke, K. (n.d.). *Getting rid of the guilt after postpartum depression*. Postpartum Progress. https://postpartumprogress.com/getting-rid-of-the-guilt-after-postpartum-depression

Kuhl, P. K. (2010). Brain mechanisms in early language acquisition. *Neuron, 67*(5), 713–727. https://doi.org/10.1016/j.neuron.2010.08.038

La Leche League International. (n.d.). *Vitamin D, your baby, and you*. https://llli.org/breastfeeding-info/vitamin-d/#:~:

Learning your baby's cues. (n.d.). Parent Club. https://www.parentclub.scot/articles/learning-your-babys-cues

Levine, H. (2022, August 28). *Vaginal delivery recovery.* WebMD. https://www. webmd.com/parenting/baby/recovery-vaginal-delivery

Lindberg, S. (2020a, January 27). *The best postpartum exercises to do right now.* Healthline. https://www.healthline.com/health/exercise-fitness/post natal-exercises#sample-workout

Lindberg, S. (2020b, July 31). *Postpartum diet plan: Tips for healthy eating after giving birth.* Healthline. https://www.healthline.com/health/postpar tum-diet

March of Dimes. (n.d.-a). *Postpartum depression.* https://www.marchofdimes. org/find-support/topics/postpartum/postpartum-depression#:~

March of Dimes. (n.d.-b). *Your body after baby: The first 6 weeks.* https://www. marchofdimes.org/find-support/topics/postpartum/your-body-after-baby-first-6-weeks

Martinez, N. A. (2024, January 31). *Create the ideal environment for the best sleep ever.* CNET. https://www.cnet.com/health/sleep/create-the-perfect-environment-for-the-best-sleep/

Mayo Clinic Staff. (2022a, August 3). *Exercise and stress: Get moving to manage stress.* Mayo Clinic. https://www.mayoclinic.org/healthy-lifestyle/ stress-management/in-depth/exercise-and-stress/art-20044469#:~

Mayo Clinic Staff. (2022b, June 4). *Breast self-exam for breast awareness.* Mayo Clinic. https://www.mayoclinic.org/tests-procedures/breast-exam/about/ pac-20393237

Mayo Clinic Staff. (2022c, November 24). *Postpartum depression.* Mayo Clinic. https://www.mayoclinic.org/diseases-conditions/postpartum-depression/ symptoms-causes/syc-20376617

Mayo Clinic Staff. (2022d, November 24). *Postpartum depression.* Mayo Clinic. https://www.mayoclinic.org/diseases-conditions/postpartum-depression/diagnosis-treatment/drc-20376623#:~

Mayo Clinic Staff. (2023, December 27). *Postpartum care: What to expect after a vaginal birth.* Mayo Clinic. https://www.mayoclinic.org/healthy-life style/labor-and-delivery/in-depth/postpartum-care/art-20047233

Mayo Clinic Staff. (2024, March 13). *Exercise after pregnancy: How to get started.* Mayo Clinic. https://www.mayoclinic.org/healthy-lifestyle/labor-and-delivery/in-depth/exercise-after-pregnancy/art-20044596

Mehta, P. (2022, April 12). *What to know about staying hydrated while pregnant and breastfeeding.* WebMD. https://www.webmd.com/baby/what-to-know-staying-hydrated-while-pregnant-breastfeeding

Migala, J. (2023, August 18). *8 permanent body changes after pregnancy.*

Health. https://www.health.com/condition/pregnancy/body-changes-post-pregnancy

Miller, L. (n.d.). *10 tips for balancing motherhood and your career.* Kindred Bravely. https://www.kindredbravely.com/blogs/bravely/balancing-moth erhood-and-career

Mind. (2022, March). *Signs and symptoms of stress.* https://www.mind.org.uk/ information-support/types-of-mental-health-problems/stress/signs-and-symptoms-of-stress/

Mindful Staff. (2020, July 8). *What is mindfulness?* Mindful. https://www. mindful.org/what-is-mindfulness/

MomMed Official. (2023, December 26). *Importance of a support system for new moms: Why it matters.* MomMed. https://mommed.com/en-gb/blogs/ content/importance-of-a-support-system-for-new-moms-why-it-matters

Mughal, S., Azhar, Y., & Siddiqui, W. (2022). *Postpartum depression.* StatPearls Publishing. https://www.ncbi.nlm.nih.gov/books/NBK519070/#:~

Murray, D. (2021, March 31). *Caring for your breasts when breastfeeding.* Verywell Family. https://www.verywellfamily.com/how-to-care-for-your-nurs ing-breasts-431863

National Institute of Health. (n.d.). *When breastfeeding, how many calories should moms and babies consume?* https://www.nichd.nih.gov/health/ topics/breastfeeding/conditioninfo/calories

Nemours KidsHealth. (n.d.). *Pregnant or breastfeeding? Nutrients you need.* https://kidshealth.org/en/parents/moms-nutrients.html

Newborn behaviour: An overview. (2022, December 20). raisingchil-dren.net.au. https://raisingchildren.net.au/newborns/behaviour/under standing-behaviour/newborn-behaviour#:~

Newton-Wellesley Hospital. (n.d.-a). *Postpartum diet and weight loss.* https:// www.nwh.org/maternity-guide/postpartum-guide/postpartum-chapter-2/ diet-and-weight-loss#:Newton-Wellesley Hospital. (n.d.-b). *Postpartum emotional adjustments.* https://www.nwh.org/maternity-guide/postpar tum-guide/postpartum-chapter-2/postpartum-emotional-adjustments

NHS. (n.d.). *Breastfeeding and diet.* National Health Service. https://www. nhs.uk/conditions/baby/breastfeeding-and-bottle-feeding/breastfeeding-and-lifestyle/diet/

Nipple care for breastfeeding mums. (n.d.). Medela. https://www.medela.com/ en/breastfeeding-pumping/articles/nipple-care-for-breastfeeding-mums

Office on Women's Health. (2023, October 13). *Postpartum depression.* U.S. Department of Health and Human Services. https://www.womenshealth. gov/mental-health/mental-health-conditions/postpartum-depression

Pacheco, D. (2023, August 10). *Understanding sleep deprivation and new parenthood.* Sleep Foundation. https://www.sleepfoundation.org/sleep-deprivation/parents

Panwar, N. (n.d.). Quote in Gillis, D. (2021, May 17). *12 uplifting quotes for moms that will make you smile.* Faith Heritage at Home. https://faithheritageathome.com/2021/05/17/12-uplifting-quotes-for-moms-that-will-make-you-smile/

Parker, H. (2022, November 24). *12 super-foods for new moms.* WebMD. https://www.webmd.com/parenting/baby/breast-feeding-diet

Pevzner, H. (2022, August 5). *A guide to your postpartum vagina.* Parents. https://www.parents.com/pregnancy/my-body/postpartum/8-ways-to-make-your-vag-feel-better-after-birth/

Playtime with your baby: Learning and growing in the first year. (2022, July). Caring for Kids. https://caringforkids.cps.ca/handouts/behavior-and-development/playtime_with_your_baby

Postpartum stress syndrome. (2023, January 16). Majka. https://lovemajka.com/blogs/blog/postpartum-stress-syndrome

Pregnancy, Birth and Baby. (n.d.). *Bonding with your baby.* https://www.pregnancybirthbaby.org.au/bonding-with-your-baby

Reed, J. (n.d.). *How new moms can get more postpartum sleep.* NewYork-Presbyterian. https://healthmatters.nyp.org/how-new-moms-can-get-more-sleep/

Rodriguez, E. (2023, March 14). *7 ways motherhood changes you.* Reader's Digest. https://www.readersdigest.co.uk/inspire/life/7-ways-motherhood-changes-you

Rowley, C. (n.d.). Quote in Shutterfly Staff. (2020, June 8). *35+ new mom quotes and words of encouragement for mothers.* Shutterfly. https://www.shutterfly.com/ideas/new-mom-quotes/

Salzer, E. B., Meireles, J. F. F., Toledo, A. F. Â., de Siqueira, M. R., Ferreira, M. E. C., & Neves, C. M. (2023). Body image assessment tools in pregnant women: A systematic review. *International Journal of Environmental Research and Public Health, 20*(3), 2258. https://doi.org/10.3390/ijerph20032258

Schroeder, W. (2024, February 16). *Breaking the chains: Exercise as a key treatment for depression.* Just Mind. https://justmind.org/breaking-the-chains-exercise-as-a-key-treatment-for-depression/

Shiraz, Z. (2023, August 18). *Mindfulness tips for new moms: Ways to deal effectively with postpartum phase.* Hindustan Times. https://www.hindustantimes.com/lifestyle/health/mindfulness-tips-for-new-moms-ways-to-deal-effectively-with-postpartum-phase-101692364353869.html

6 body changes after pregnancy. (n.d.). HealthXchange.sg. https://www. healthxchange.sg/wellness/physical-health/body-changes-after-preg nancy

6 ways to handle postpartum stress. (n.d.). Green Valley OBGYN. https:// gvobgyn.com/ways-to-handle-postpartum-stress/

Stewart, R. (2023, December 21). *How to play with your baby.* Parents. https:// www.parents.com/baby/development/the-best-ways-to-play-with-your-baby/

Styler, T. (n.d.). *Trudie Styler quotes.* BrainyQuote. https://www.brainyquote. com/quotes/trudie_styler_865046

Suni, E., & Rehman, A. (2023, November 8). *How to design the ideal bedroom for sleep.* Sleep Foundation. https://www.sleepfoundation.org/bedroom-environment/how-to-design-the-ideal-bedroom-for-sleep

Taylor, M. (2021, September 7). *The parent-baby bond: What if it doesn't happen right away?* What to Expect. https://www.whattoexpect.com/first-year/ask-heidi/week-1/postpartum-bonding.aspx

Taylor, R. B. (n.d.-a). *Baby talk: Communicating with your baby through reading, singing, and more.* WebMD. https://www.webmd.com/parenting/baby/baby-talk

Taylor, R. B. (n.d.-b). *Breast problems after breastfeeding.* WebMD. https:// www.webmd.com/parenting/baby/after-nursing

Thinking and play: Babies. (2022, December 12). Raising Children Network. https://raisingchildren.net.au/babies/play-learning/play-baby-develop ment/thinking-play-babies

3 steps to building your postpartum support network. (n.d.). Lansinoh. https:// lansinoh.com/blogs/birth-prep-recovery/3-steps-to-building-your-postpar tum-support-network

Tirtadji, B. (2019, November 21). *18 tips to create the ultimate sleep environ-ment and improve your quality of sleep.* Somnox. https://somnox.com/blog/18-tips-to-create-the-ultimate-sleep-environment-and-improve-your-quality-of-sleep/

Tommy's. (n.d.). *When and how to exercise after a c-section.* https://www. tommys.org/pregnancy-information/giving-birth/caesarean-section/when-and-how-exercise-after-c-section

Traxler, C. (2023, April 14). *Postpartum diet plan: Best foods to eat after giving birth.* Zaya Care. https://zayacare.com/blog/postpartum-diet-plan/

200 new mom quotes and words of encouragement for mothers. (2023, April

29). Blissbies. https://blissbies.com/blog/quotes-words-of-encourage ment-for-new-mothers/#:~

UnityPoint Health. (n.d.). *Postpartum vaginal care: Hygiene tips for after giving birth*. https://www.unitypoint.org/news-and-articles/postpartum-vaginal-care-hygiene-tips-for-after-giving-birth

Vitamin B12. (2024). In *Drugs and Lactation Database (LactMed®)*. National Institute of Child Health and Human Development. https://www.ncbi.nlm.nih.gov/books/NBK534419/

Waits, W. (2023, July 23). *Can you prevent postpartum depression? Strategies to reduce your risk*. Talkiatry. https://www.talkiatry.com/blog/how-to-avoid-postpartum-depression

Waller, J. (2023, May 4). *6 easy postpartum yoga poses for birth recovery*. Motherly. https://www.mother.ly/health-wellness/fitness/easy-postpartum-yoga/

Wati, L. R., Sargowo, D., Nurseta, T., & Zuhriyah, L. (2023). The role of protein intake on the total milk protein in lead-exposed lactating mothers. *Nutrients*, *15*(11), 2584. https://doi.org/10.3390/nu15112584

Watson, E. (n.d.). *Emma Watson quotes*. AZ Quotes. https://www.azquotes.com/quote/814386

WebMD Editorial Contributors. (n.d.). *Understanding postpartum depression—diagnosis and treatment*. WebMD. https://www.webmd.com/depression/postpartum-depression/understanding-postpartum-depression-treat ment

Weiss, K. (2021, October 5). *How to talk to your baby*. What to Expect. https://www.whattoexpect.com/first-year/milestones/how-to-talk-to-babies

Why it's so normal to feel emotional after childbirth—and when to get help. (n.d.). Bodily. https://itsbodily.com/blogs/birth-recovery-postpartum/post partum-emotions-changes-after-giving-birth

Zamosky, L. (n.d.). *5 new mom guilt trips to skip*. WebMD. https://www.webmd.com/parenting/baby/features/new-mom-guilt

56764599R00109